ORTHOPAEDIC SURGEON | RESEARCHER | TEAM DOC

DR. VONDA WRIGHT'S

GUIDE TO THRIVE

FOUR STEPS TO
Body, Brains,
and **Bliss**

VONDA WRIGHT, M.D.

Library of Congress Cataloging-in-Publication Data

Wright, Vonda.
    Dr. Vonda Wright's guide to THRIVE : four steps to body, brains, and bliss / Vonda Wright.
        p. cm.
    ISBN 978-1-60078-599-3
    1. Exercise for middle-aged persons. 2. Physical fitness for middle-aged persons. 3. Middle-aged persons—Health and hygiene. 4. Middle-aged persons—Mental health. I. Title.
    GV482.6.W748 2011
    613.70446—dc23

                        2011025256

This book is available in quantity at special discounts for your group or organization. For further information, contact:

TRIUMPH BOOKS
542 South Dearborn Street
Suite 750
Chicago, Illinois 60605
(312) 939–3330
Fax (312) 663–3557
www.triumphbooks.com

Printed in U.S.A.
ISBN: 978-1-60078-599-3
Design by Paul Petrowsky

Photography credits. 1. Peter Taglianetti: Two-time Stanley Cup champion and fitness expert www.petertags.com
2. Duane Reider: Duane Reider Photography, Pittsburgh, PA www.duanereiderphotography.com
3. Thrive exercise equipment demonstrated in this book sold exclusively at Dick's Sporting Goods Stores
4. iStock photos as indicated

CONTENTS

Love and all my best to

Isabella
my pure joy and bliss who motivates
what I really want out of life,

Mom
who taught me strength and courage
and is now teaching my daughter,

Dad
who dazzles me and everyone he meets
with his love of life

Collin
who perseveres in building a thriving life

Peter
the rock who gives me amazing advice,
support, and partnership

Acknowledgments

As a surgeon, mother, daughter, and author I have had the extraordinary opportunity to listen and learn from amazing people throughout my life and career. Sometimes they are the giants in their fields, my patients as they teach me about themselves or long-abiding friends.

Once again, my first thanks go to God and my family. To God for giving me a mind capable of invention, the hands to create, and the stamina to get it all done. To my family, Gene, Joy, and Collin Wright, unending gratitude for being a solid foundation and support for my vision. I am again most thankful for wondrous Isabella. Spending my life watching her grow would be enough.

I thank the hundreds of fascinating and inspiring masters athletes and "Starters" who motivate me to change the way we age in this country. In them I see the real-life examples of how a daily conscious decision to invest in oneself manifests in Body, Brains, and Bliss. I am thankful they take the time to participate in my research.

For bringing *Guide to THRIVE* out of my office and into the world I thank Triumph Books and my literary agent, Steve Mandell. Specifically, I am thankful that president Mitch Rogatz and editorial director Tom Bast believed in my vision. I am thankful to the Triumph team: Don Gulbrandsen, managing editor, and Karen O'Brien, associate editor, for their countless hours in expertly managing the details of the manuscript preparation, and Natalie King and Fred Walski for charging forth with PR and marketing. Thanks also to Rex Halbeisen and Kevin Dill of Connect U Marketing for their web creativity. To Robin Waxenberg, last but certainly not least amongst this group, thanks for her tireless pursuit of the media and championing my platform.

Special thanks to Peter Taglianetti, two-time Stanley Cup champion and fitness expert (petertags.com) for agreeing to demonstrate the "moves" in this book as well as the patience to give solid advice as I bounced ideas off him, and for the creative eye of Duane Reider, our photographer, (duanereiderphotography.com) thanks for capturing my words in pictures.

Finally, I am thankful to the giants on whose shoulders I stand. I have had the great fortune to learn from some of the best experts throughout my career about orthopaedic surgery but most importantly about life. Some of their wisdom I have shared with you in this book.

Writing *Guide to THRIVE* redoubled my passion for changing the way we age in this country. It was motivated by the lives and stories of the people I am privileged to care for in my clinics, the O.R., and on the playing field. I realize that by helping and motivating people to maintain mobility throughout their life spans that we can actually save their lives and lifestyles. For a job that lets me do this, I am thankful.

My best to you.
Vonda Wright, MD

Introduction

"The purpose of life is to live it, to taste experience to the utmost, to reach out eagerly and without fear for newer and richer experience."
—Eleanor Roosevelt

These are the best years of your life! No matter what stage of life you are in, you can make this year the beginning of your best years. Look in the mirror: strong, smart, happy, and in control…you are not a kid anymore!

Not happy with what you see?
You can see it with my four practical steps for THRIVING:
A Vision, Action, Attitude, and Achieve

No one wants to just get by or merely survive another day, but that's where we can sometimes find ourselves if we are not purposeful about how we are living. Living healthy, vital, joyful, and THRIVING lives is an active and intentional process.

Guide to THRIVE is based on my extensive work with masters athletes and adult onset exercisers who have literally changed their lives by paying attention to the lifestyle choices they make. I have seen everyday people—people who were stuck in a track toward middle-age with seemingly nowhere to go but old—change their bodies, their brains, and the way they feel about themselves, their lives, and the future….bliss. I translate practical advice into real-life action using tactics learned as a surgeon, sports doctor, thinker, businesswoman, athlete, mother of a three-year-old, and the head of a household.

THRIVE-ing is intentional, fun, a lot of work, and not always easy. I share stories of encouragement from my own life and the lives of the people I am honored to care for. I also pass along the real-life advice I have received from the giants who have mentored me. As an academic surgeon, I insist on the best information backed up by solid research. Your Body, Brain, and Bliss connection is not just opinion but good science.

Guide to THRIVE is divided into four sections. Section 1 unfolds by preparing you for six remarkable months of Body, Brains, and Bliss transformation using four practical steps. You learn steps for creating **A Vision** for your future: "What do you really want, and where are you going?" We take **Action** by assessing our physical health, fitness level, and current nutrition. We then apply your plan to your **Attitude** by learning about the science of the Body, Brains, and Bliss connection, assessing where we are now and what the barriers have been to THRIV-ing. By the end of Section 1, we are ready to **Achieve** and set specific six-month goals for your Body, Brains, and Bliss.

Sections 2, 3, and 4 are each two-month seasons of A Vision, Action, Attitude, and Achieve. Each section builds on the last and supplies vital guidance on self-assessment and how to have a THRIVE-ing Body by MOVE-ing and EAT-ing. I've designed specific weekly exercise and nutrition guides that first lead you through a total body fitness program and then teach you how to design the program that is right for you. This gives you control over your goals.

I also teach you about the fascinating physical connection between exercise, your Body, and how your Brain thinks and feels. Each two-month season provides you with practical exercises and tools for keeping our Attitude strong and sharp. Each section concludes by evaluating our Achievement in the previous two months and making Action plans for the next two months.

Guide to THRIVE is not just a book. I have written it as if you are sitting across from me in my office, at a dinner party, or at the gym. I invite you to join my amazing *Guide to THRIVE F.A.N.* (Fitness And Nutrition) Club. It is like having your very own private consultation. You will enter your own health, fitness, and nutrition information and in return receive health-risk assessment information specific to you as well as fitness and nutrition tips tailored to you.

Your *Guide to THRIVE* does not end on the last page. Throughout the book you will notice QR barcodes. These are immediate portals from your smart phone to more information, exercise videos, and personal encouragement from me.

In the midst of a full life, you can THRIVE by having A Vision, taking Action, changing your Attitude, and Achieving the life you dream about.

I am excited for you.

These are the best years.

This is the year you will THRIVE!

① Prepare to THRIVE

"Go confidently in the direction of your dreams! Live the life you've imagined."

—Henry David Thoreau, *Walden*

CHAPTER 1

Preparing A Vision for Your Life

"The tragedy in life doesn't lie in not reaching your goal. The tragedy lies in having no goal to reach."

—Benjamin May

THRIVE-ing is about adding high-quality years to your life, not just passing the time. Just think of it. You have the power to make your life healthy, vital, active, and joyful. The first step down this path is knowing where you are going.

Figuring out what you want your life to look like is not easy, but as Andy Stanley said in *Visioneering*, "Vision gives significance to otherwise meaningless details of our lives."

For most of us, it is not dreaming the impossible dream, but it is a realistic picture of what you want your life to be. It is a reflection of your values, why you exist, and what you want to become.

No matter where you are in life—just starting out of college, raising your children, getting the 20-year watch at work, or thinking about what to do during your empty-nest years—creating A Vision will motivate, inspire, and direct your path.

I learned a big lesson about Vision-casting early in my career. As I was training I always said I wanted to someday be the chairman of the department. I'm not sure why but I was an ambitious academic surgeon, so it seemed like a star to reach for. Starting an academic surgical practice is not easy, with long hours, sick patients, trying to prove myself, write grants, publish research, etc. We call it "gunning."

One day, I was at a hospital event talking to a plastic surgeon we call the Pizza Man. The Pizza Man is an amazing surgeon, and no matter how bad things are or what time of the day or night they happen, we knew if we called him, he always delivered. As residents we often wondered why he worked like that at such great personal sacrifice.

That night, I was groaning about how hard all the years of gunning were and the political roadblocks in my way. At that point, he taught me one of the most important lessons I have ever learned. After listening to me whine, he simply looked at me and said, "Vonda, what I can tell you is that if you just figure out what's *most* important to you, everything else will fall into place."

At first I didn't get it, but then it dawned on me. He worked like he did because he liked being the one who delivers under all circumstances, no matter what. It is his motivation, his passion, and it makes the sacrifices no sacrifice to him.

For me, figuring out what I really wanted from life didn't mean I had to choose the same path as my mentors. I learned that casting a Vision for my life meant THRIVE-ing both inside and outside the hospital. I have broad interests, and they take a lot of energy. However, because I know my Vision, gunning is not painful at all.

In this chapter we will take the time to look at what you want from life, where you are going, and what THRIVE-ing means to you. The goal is to move you toward a destination of your choice—not merely unintentionally moving forward.

Step 1 is realizing you need an overall Vision for your life. Step 2 is getting to know you.

When you are dating and getting to know someone or even developing a new business relationship, it's all about taking the time to notice people and knowing where they are now and where they want to be in the future.

Creating a Vision for your life begins the same way. When was the last time you really stopped to notice yourself? What do you look like? What do you spend the most time thinking about? What do you value the most? How do you work? What motivates you? What is the state of your relationships?

Set some time aside to gather some information about yourself by answering these questions:

1. What are your abilities? What are you naturally good at, not just what you have learned to do?

2. What is your personality? Are you an extrovert, introvert? Is the glass half-full or half-empty?

3. What skills have you acquired over the years?

4. What types of things interest you? What are you passionate about?

5. What do you value? Reputation, hard work, family time, quiet time, a strong body?

6. What are your goals for life, your body, brains, bliss?

7. What stage are you in life? Recent grad, raising kids, middle aged?

8. What was your family of origin like? Often this sets a tone for your life.

9. What did your last success look like?

10. When was the last time you were fit?

11. Are you happy? When was the last time you were truly happy?

Step 3 in casting your Vision is creating an umbrella statement for why you are building a personal vision statement. These may look like, "I want to live a healthy, joyful, connected life," or, "While climbing the corporate ladder, I want to balance my professional and personal life," or "I want to raise happy, healthy, kind children."

Your building blocks for achieving your Vision are the tools, values, and desires you listed in step 2. Step 4 is to pull the most important elements you want to have going forward from the lists you created above and write them under your umbrella statement.

Step 5 is to take a stab at writing a statement. This is not the final product, and I predict your Vision statement will go through a lot of permutations before it is settled in your mind. This is an important exercise even if you never perfect it because it will stay in your mind as you frame your life day to day. Here is an example of one of several of my early stabs at Vision casting:

"I will maximize my good hands and talent for teaching and communicating to change the paradigm of aging in this country."

"I will stop disorganized 'bricklaying' in order to maximize the time I spend with my daughter."

"I will work to get into the best physical, mental, and emotional shape of my life."

You can find many examples and tools online to assist in this process. These are some more examples I found:

Personal Mission Statement Template Sample:
My mission is to use my [passion/abilities/positive personality traits] to achieve [goals] based on my [principle/values].

Step 6 is to walk away from the writing. Take some time to mull over all these lists you have made and the draft statement you wrote to imagine what living your statement means. What does your life look like if you live the life you've envisioned?

What does an ideal day at work look like? How is your day arranged? What does your body look and feel like? What are you thinking about? What are your relationships like with your family and/or children? How do you feel about your life?

If you normally use your imagination, thinking through these questions will be easy for you. If you are normally a very concrete and logistical thinker, like I am, this may be a stretch. However, it's an important stretch to complement the list-making we just did.

The last step before you cast A Vision for your life is to talk about this process with someone who knows you. This will help you consolidate the lists of personal attributes you made while thinking it through by communication.

When you are ready, write down your Vision. In this book I teach you tools to THRIVE through MOVE-ing, EAT-ing, THINK-ing, and FEEL-ing. Your vision will give significance to the details.

Now, let's MOVE!

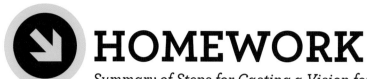

HOMEWORK

Summary of Steps for Casting a Vision for your Life

1. Answer these questions:

    a. What are your abilities? What are you naturally good at?,

    b. What is your personality? Are you an extrovert or an introvert? Are you positive or negative?

    c. What skills have you acquired over the years?

    d. What types of things interest you? What are you passionate about?

    e. What do you value?

    f. What are your goals for your life, your body, your brains, and your bliss?

    g. What stage are you in life?

    h. What was your family like?

    i. What did your last success look like?

    j. When was the last time you were fit?

    k. Are you happy? When was the last time you were truly happy?

2. Create an umbrella Vision statement.

    a. Write the most important elements you want to include in your Vision from the list you made in step 2.

    b. Write a draft Vision statement.

    c. Take time to visualize what this statement looks like in life and what it means to you.

    d. Talk over this process with someone who knows you.

3. Cast a Vision for your future and write it down.

NOTES

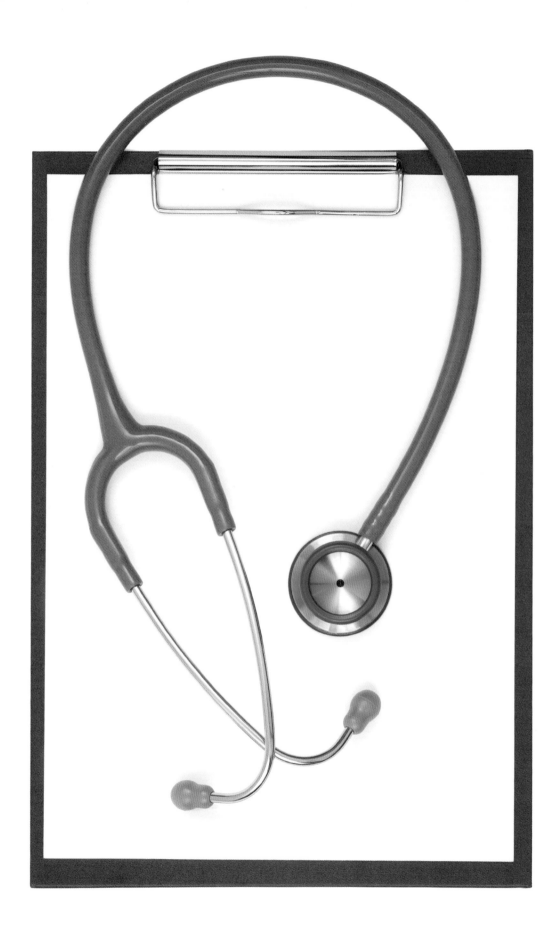

CHAPTER 2

Prepare to Take ACTION: Become an Expert...On Yourself

"To keep the body in good health is a duty. Otherwise we shall not be able to keep our mind strong and clear."
—**Buddha**

In the last chapter you did a lot of thinking about a Vision for your life. In this chapter you make the next step by taking Action for your Body. Here, I set you up to THRIVE by MOVE-ing and EAT-ing. You can't know where you are going unless you know your starting point. So become an expert...on yourself.

▶ HEALTH = PLEASURE,
so Take Time to Rewire your Brain

Before we start, I want you to set up a reward to give yourself if you do all the work in this chapter—not a big jelly donut but a small event, a little luxury, such as a call to an old friend you miss. I am big into small rewards for achieving short-term goals. This not only helps us rewire our brain to associate healthy habits with pleasure (instead of viewing them as work), but it also gives us something to look forward to. For instance, my reward for finishing this chapter is to take my daughter to kindermusic, which is pure pleasure.

My reward for "Getting to know myself" is:

▶ KNOW YOUR BODY

Your first step is to get to know your physical body. Go stand in front of the mirror. It's okay.

What physical traits do you like the most? Do you have amazing eyes, long legs, strong back, great posture? Write down what you see here:

What physical traits would you like to work on? Are you too apple-shaped, do you have weak buttocks, or are you tired of your hair color? Write down the areas you prioritize here:

▶ KNOW YOUR NUMBERS

Next, it's time to know your numbers. What happens on the outside of your body says a lot about what is going on inside.

I encourage my patients to carry a card with these numbers in their wallets or log them into their smartphone of choice.

	Today	Comments
Weight		
Height		
Waist		Measure just below your navel. Ideally, women < 35 inches, men < 40 inches
Hip		Measure just above your hip bones
Waist/Hip Ratio (Divide your waist measurement by hip measurement)		Ideal is < 0.8, the closer to 1.0, the higher your health risks
Resting Heart Rate		Measure first thing in the morning or after sitting quietly for 15 minutes
Maximum Heart Rate		
Obtain these values from a visit to your doctor's office		
Cholesterol		
Triglycerides		
LDL		
HDL		
Fasting Blood Glucose		
Blood Pressure		120/80 is normal
Percent Body Fat		

PREPARE TO TAKE ACTION: BECOME AN EXPERT...ON YOURSELF

▶ EVEN HEALTHY PEOPLE NEED A DOCTOR

Ideally, the first time you have a serious illness is not the first time you want to meet your doctor. Every healthy adult should establish a relationship with a primary care physician.

Keep the following medical history items together in a file and take them to your doctor's visit. These are the questions he or she will ask you:

1. Today's specific symptoms
   a. When did they start?
   b. What do they feel like?
   c. What makes them better/worse?
   d. What have you taken to treat them?
2. Past Medical History
   a. What health problems have you been treated for in the past (including childhood)? Think through every body system, including:
      i. Head/neck
      ii. Heart/BP
      iii. Lungs
      iv. GI system (stomach, intestines, liver, pancreas)
      v. Musculoskeletal
      vi. Metabolic (diabetes, thyroid, adrenal)
      vii. GU system (kidneys, gyne organs)
      viii. Infectious diseases
3. Past Surgical History
   a. What surgeries have you had in the past? When did they occur, and who performed them?
4. Allergies
   a. Medications

b. Food

c. Know the reaction that occurred

5. Current Medications

    a. Prescription

        i. Dose and frequency

    b. Over the counter

    c. Supplements

6. Immunizations

7. Social history

    a. Tobacco

        i. Do you smoke now?

        ii. Did you ever smoke?

        iii. How many packs per day for how many years?

8. Family History

    a. What illnesses occur in your family?

        i. Mother/father/siblings

        ii. Grandparents

        iii. Aunts/uncles

        iv . If they are deceased, what age did they die and of what cause?

Pay special attention to heart attack, blood pressure, stroke, diabetes, cancer, and metabolic disease.

Go to my website, www.vondawright.com, to print tables of the prevention tests your doctor should obtain for you for each decade. They are a great way to keep up with health maintenance.

In today's atmosphere of health care uncertainty, I teach my patients to take more responsibility for their health and know their own health history. Who can know you better than yourself?

▶ JOIN THE THRIVE F.A.N. CLUB

My THRIVE Fitness And Nutrition (F.A.N.) Club is an amazing interactive online tool that uses your own numbers, the ones you just gathered, to provide you with an individualized health profile. This is not a generic set of instructions but is all about you specifically.

By answering the 78 health assessment questions online, the F.A.N. Club will tell you what diseases you are at risk for and give you specific tips for minimizing your risks. It provides important questions to review with your physician, as well.

In addition, the F.A.N. club also provides the following amazing components:

✓ **Health Tracker:** Keep track of your numbers digitally and update them to follow your progress.

✓ **Nutrition Assessment:** Determine what are you eating now and how it measures up to what your body needs. You will receive specific tips for making small changes for healthier EAT-ing.

✓ **Fitness Assessment:** The F.A.N. Club takes you through several specific tests of flexibility, strength, and endurance that measure your baseline fitness and predict your health level. You will receive specific tips for making your first MOVE.

✓ **Fitness Tracker with Cardio Log:** This is an additional tool to track your daily workouts.

You can register for this amazing resource on my website at www.vondawright.com or by using your smartphone to scan the QR link.

▶ TAKING ACTION FOR YOUR BODY:
MOVE-ing and EAT-ing

The word *doctor* is derived from a word meaning *teacher*, and that is what I really am. Sure, I perform surgery several days per week, but the greatest amount of my time is spent teaching my patients about their injuries, their bodies, and their health. Together we make Action plans that change their lives. My goal is always to teach them so well that they become independent and can teach others what they have learned.

This is my goal for you, too. Each two-month Action section builds on the last, and at the end of six months, you are equipped to THRIVE on your own.

Here is what to expect:

Months 1–2:

Making the First MOVE

I teach you how to MOVE via short Total Body THRIVE (TBT) exercises and circuits focusing on aerobic exercise and carrying a load.

Know What You EAT

When it comes to diet, you definitely have to know yourself. I teach you the 500 rule and to watch what you eat and a few simple substitutions that mean big change.

Months 3–4:

Keep MOVE-ing to F.A.C.E. Your Future

Maximizing performance and minimizing injury requires attention to the four components of fitness. I expand your TBT circuits by adding flexibility and equilibrium/balance circuits to the aerobic exercise and carrying a load you learned in the first two months.

Know Your Food

Eating well isn't rocket science, but it is hard to make good decisions if you don't know what your body needs. I teach you about your foods—the good, the bad, and the ugly.

Months 5–6:

Show Me Your Own MOVE-s

Now that you are equipped with a large menu of TBT exercises, I now teach you how to design your own circuits and create exercise independence.

Planning Ahead to EAT Well

Your body has a waistline, not a waste line. It takes a little planning to give your body what it needs and not give in to fast food. Here I teach you how to plan well and give you examples of how I do it.

▶ SAFETY FIRST *with the PAR-Q*

If you are not a consistent exerciser, it is safest to answer the following questions to assess your risk for starting a new exercise program. If you answer any of the following questions with a "YES," see your doctor prior to beginning to MOVE.

1. Has your doctor ever said that you have a heart condition and that you should do only physical activity recommended by a doctor?

2. Do you feel pain in your chest when you do physical activity?

3. In the past month, have you had chest pain when you were not doing physical activity?

4. Do you lose your balance because of dizziness, or do you ever lose consciousness?

5. Do you have a bone or joint problem that could be made worse by a change in your physical activity?

6. Is your doctor currently prescribing drugs for your blood pressure or heart condition?

▶ MAKE AN EXCUSE LIST

I'm about to give you permission to make excuses for why you have not taken Action to invest in your health daily. Now's your chance, and I want to hear them. I understand the fullness of the lives we lead, being pulled in 20 directions, being busy with family and financial obligations. I have made these excuses myself, and I have heard them all before from my patients. Some are really logical, while others are just plain silly. Write them down now so they are out in the open and we can take action to excuse the excuses!

▶ **TELL EVERYONE** *You are Taking Action to THRIVE!*

You are more likely to stick with a plan if you are held accountable by your friends. When I am going to run a big race, I have to keep myself accountable to train by actually paying the money and registering for the race far ahead of time, then I tell everybody in my life I'm going to do it. It becomes a topic of conversation—people ask me about it, and some people even end up joining me.

Think of at least five people you are going to tell about your plans and then tell them. Ask them to join you. If you belong to a book club, get everyone involved. What better way to enrich your lives than by THRIVE-ing together? (If you need something literary to discuss, use the quotes at the beginning of the chapters.)

List the five people who will keep you accountable.

Taking Action and becoming an expert on yourself is a lot of work, and you deserve that little reward you chose at the beginning of this chapter. Before you reward yourself, however, go for a walk. Right now. Take 10 or 15 minutes just for yourself, leave your phone behind, breathe deep, and walk. What better way to take Action for your body than to make a MOVE right now.

When you get back we will learn why your little walk probably made you smarter.

Now MOVE.

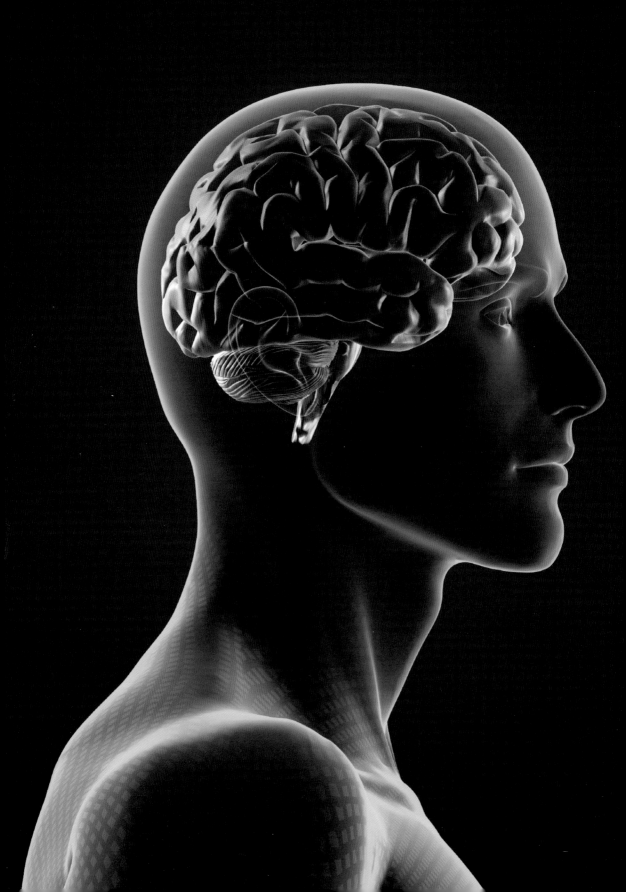

CHAPTER 3

Prepare Your Attitude: Build a Better Brain

"The more fit you are, the more resilient your brain becomes and the better it functions both cognitively and psychologically. If you get your body in shape, your mind will follow."

—John Ratey, M.D. Spark

So far you have prepared to THRIVE by creating a Vision for your future, and you have taken Action by critically assessing where your Body is starting from on this six-month journey. Now it's time to focus on your Attitude.

For the purposes of THRIVE-ing, your Attitude includes how your Brain Thinks and how you feel, or what I've called Bliss. Your Body, Brains, and Bliss are vitally connected, and all three must be healthy to truly THRIVE.

The good news is that your Body, Brains, and Bliss are not only figuratively connected but physically connected. This connection first hit me when I was sitting in a research meeting of the geriatrics department at UPMC. They were presenting some of their work, using an MRI technique, documenting that the same areas of the brain that were active during exercise were also active during cognitive thinking and also when the person was feeling emotion. Many other exciting studies support this connection between our Body, Brains, and Bliss and give us a common tool for THRIVE-ing in our physical, mental, and emotional health. That wonder tool is exercise.

The fact is, it's no wonder at all that exercise strengthens the brain's ability to learn. Even at a cellular level, we are wired for mobility. Chronic intense activity increases capillary development in the brain, enabling oxygen, glucose, and a spectrum of growth hormones access to the brain. In addition, our bodies respond to the physical stress of exercise as if we were trying to escape danger—the old flight-or-fight mechanism. When we get our blood pumping, under real stress or stress induced by running in the park, we release norepinephrine, or adrenaline and we stimulate the endocannabinoid system in our brains. Adrenaline acts on the brain to sharpen our attention, increase our arousal, and motivate us to assimilate new information, or learn. At the same time, serotonin is released to calm the brain's "nerves" so we can think straight. This puts our brain in a prime environment for learning. For many years the adrenaline camp has received all the credit for the Brain/Bliss connection to exercise. Research published in 2003 by the Georgia Institute of Technology, however, found that the sense of well-being, stress reduction, pain relief, and even that "floaty" feeling post-exercise was due to the release of molecules called endocannabinoids. These molecules, made by the exercising body, act on the brain in a similar way that smoking marijuana does and leaves us feeling the post-exercise Bliss. Exercise is the wonder tool for connecting our Body, Brains, and Bliss in the short term. Since the early 1990s, neuroscientists have known that exercise increases the release of a neurotrophin, or brain-derived neurotrophic factor (BDNF). BDNF "fertilizes" existing neurons to function better and stimulates the growth of new nerve cells for long-term brain health. And all this comes from just a little run in the park.

▶ THE BODY-BRAIN CONNECTION:
The Science Behind a Healthy Brain

I get so excited thinking about how smart and calm we are all going to be when we start using the mobility wonder tool that I wouldn't blame you if you put this book down and took a break for a run in the park right now! No matter what your age or skill level, getting off the couch and onto the playground has a profound effect on the brain's structure and function.

Studies have found that the brains of active children have more developed centers for cognitive function than those of sedentary kids. Beckman and Kramer of the University of Illinois used MRIs to look at the brains of these two groups. They found the hippocampus, a part of the brain responsible for reasoning and thinking, was 12 percent bigger in the active kids than the sedentary group. This translated into improved scores of memory and information integration.

Researchers at USC reported that better cardiovascular health among teenage boys correlated to higher intelligence test scores, more education, and ultimately more income later in life. Using the Swedish population registry, scientists found performance on all measures of cognitive function increased directly with the level of aerobic fitness.

There are parts of brain development and function that kids can't do anything about, such as genetics and socioeconomic status. But exercising is an easy and free way to physically give our kids' brains the best shot.

Kids' brains aren't the only lucky benefactor of exercise, however. Once adults hit the age of 40, we begin to lose about five percent of our brain volume per decade—and our brain actually shrinks! By 70 this process accelerates. Not only does the brain get lighter, but the creation of new brain cells, or neurons, drops. Are you feeling light-headed?

The good news is that for adults of all ages, even a single episode of intense exercise promotes the release of BDNF for the brain. In mice, exercise improves the production of brain stem cells by 200 percent.

Approximately 70 to 80 percent of BDNF is made in the brain and is important for neuron production and repair. Gold and associates found that a single 30-minute session of moderate exercise resulted in a significant increase in blood BDNF. Vega's group found the same effect with 10 minutes of intense activity.

Dr. John Ratey suggests maximizing the benefits of exercise on thinking by combining physical exertion—which expands the capillaries, builds and traffics growth factors, and stimulates cell growth—with an activity that challenges your brain, thus requiring it to make complex neural connections in order to play. Multiple other fascinating studies support the need for intense exercise to produce the most brain food.

Multiple studies also show activity can not only prevent but treat cognitive decline in the healthy and in the cognitively impaired. Researchers at the Mayo Clinic observed a cross-section of more than 1,000 octogenarians and found that those who participated in moderate exercise during mid to late life were 39 percent less likely to develop dementia. This may be due to the abundance of small blood vessels and improved cerebral blood flow found in the brains of active agers by researchers at UNC using 3D MRI scans.

An interventional study by colleagues at the University of Pittsburgh found a six-month program of intense exercise caused subjects to learn faster and achieve greater brain blood flow than the sedentary control group of middle-aged and aged participants. Dr. Baker of the University of Washington went even further to document improved cognitive ability in people who already had mild dementia after they participated in a six-month exercise program. The greatest improvements were seen in areas of executive control, such as planning, working memory, multitasking, and dealing with ambiguity.

Ratey, in his excellent book *Spark*, sums it up nicely: "The research consistently shows that the more fit you are, the more resilient your brain becomes and the better it functions both cognitively and psychologically. If you get your body in shape, your mind will follow."

▶ THE BODY-BLISS CONNECTION:
The Science Behind Exercise and Happiness

Talk to athletes, and they will tell you that even a single episode of intense exercise will make them feel better. Is this blissfulness just in their heads, or is there actually a scientific basis for promoting exercise to put you in a better mood?

Dr. Jeremy Sibold of the University of Vermont found moderate aerobic activity improves mood immediately after exercise and for up to 12 hours afterward.

Intense physical activity stimulates the production of endorphins in the brain. These chemicals are your body's own private stash of opiates, and they bind to our body's opioid receptors to block the transmission of pain signals, thus producing a euphoric feeling. This feeling doesn't happen with a leisurely walk in the park, however. When our body starts feeling the burn of moving from an easy aerobic state to a higher-demand anaerobic state, we release endorphins to ease the pain and the euphoria occurs.

Endorphins are not the only mind-altering end product of exercise. Exercise works as a holistic mood elevator, stimulating the release of adrenaline to wake up the brain; serotonin to calm the brain, decrease anxiety, and fight cortisol; and dopamine, which gives us a feeling of well-being and satisfaction; and endocannabionids, which decrease stress, pain, and anxiety.

Researchers Smitt and Otto out of Boston University explored the body of scientific studies, looking at the role of exercise and mental health. They found that people who exercise feel fewer symptoms of anxiety and depression and have lower overall stress and anger. Exercisers in the studies experienced changes in their brains' neuropathways similar to antidepressant medication. Even after short bouts of intense activity, exercise improves your mood, decreases stress levels, and makes you feel like you have more energy. The team even recommended using exercise as an addition to traditional medical therapy for depression and anxiety for everyone but especially for those people limited by the cost of or access to traditional care.

In a landmark study out of Duke University, Blumenthal and colleagues tested the idea that exercise was as effective as antidepressants for treating depression. The subjects either received antidepressant medication alone, exercise alone, or a combination of both. The depression of all three groups improved significantly, and the researchers concluded that exercise was as effective as medication in the treatment of depression and continued to be effective for more than six months.

The jury is still out as to the complete pathway between the body and mood. The Body-Bliss connection has to do not only with the chemicals released during activity but the chemical and physical pathways they travel in the brain. While scientists work hard to figure it all out, my advice—and the advice of many other experts—is just give it a try. Feeling good is just down the road.

Is feeling happy the only benefit of exercise? Absolutely not. Exercise is a great stress modulator. Stress is anything you say it is, and we all feel it differently. The things that stress me out may not be worrisome to you at all. Whatever the cause of your stress reaction, it is the healthy mode of operation for our brains, and it was designed to give our brains the tools to function during the fight-or-flight state. When we experience stress, our brains are aroused by adrenaline and focused by the release of dopamine.

When stress becomes overwhelming or chronic, however, it can start to erode the neural pathways that keep our mind connected. The continual release of stress hormones is detrimental to our brains and bodies alike. It is thought that chronic exercise decreases stress by raising the physical and mental stress threshold, elevating self-esteem, and stimulating the release of BDNF, which increases brain plasticity and neuron growth and combats the effects of chronic cortisol exposure.

While the scientific support for the connection between our Bodies, Brains, and Bliss is fascinating, building brain mass and adding bliss to our lives are both powerful incentives for getting off the couch and on the road. I hope you feel the excitement of where we are about to go. The future belongs to you.

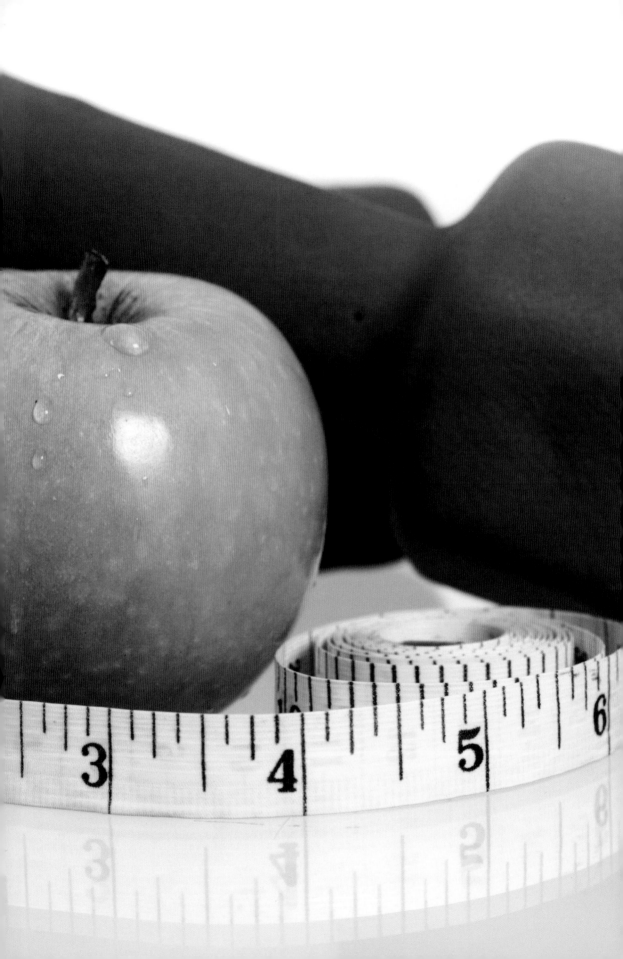

CHAPTER 4

Prepare to Achieve: See the Big Picture

"The results you achieve will be in direct proportion to the effort you apply."

—Denis Waitley, American motivational speaker

Did you do your homework? Much of my *Guide to THRIVE* involves taking the time to invest daily in yourself. Preparing to THRIVE by thinking through and doing the homework in this section is your first investment. I know sometimes—maybe even most of the time—you may be your last priority as your family, job, and friends make demands of your time. But you are worth the investment.

Now, what is the Vision you created for your future? Write it down again. I suggest, for the next six months, you put it everywhere you will see it— by your bed, in your PDA, on the bathroom mirror, near the computer at work, and in the car. It will serve as a constant reminder of what you want.

Remember that as you progress, your Vision may modify or your priorities may change. That is fine. This is not your last chance. If you need something or help from someone to accomplish your goal, don't be afraid to ask for it. Sometimes we are afraid to ask for what we want, but I have always been pleasantly surprised when I feel like I am going out on a limb to ask for something and the person says, "Yes!" After all, what is the worst thing that can happen by asking? The answer could be merely no. No harm, no foul.

Next, choose one or two people to update on your progress consistently. Talk about what you are doing each week, how it feels, and invite them to join your THRIVE-ing process. This not only keeps you accountable, but it can also serve to clarify what you are thinking as your confidants reflect back to you what you have said. Who will you choose?

The *Guide to THRIVE* is specifically equipping you to focus on your Body (MOVE-ing and EAT-ing), Brains (THINK-ing), and Bliss (FEEL-ing). I usually categorize career, business relationships, and education along with THINK-ing goals, and personal relationship, stress, happiness, etc., are grouped with FEEL-ing. Invest time now in formulating the goals you would like to Achieve in each of these four areas over the next six months and how they relate to your overall Vision for your future.

As you write, start out generally and then become very specific. In each of the next sections, we will break down these six-month goals for THRIVE-ing into smaller, more manageable two-month segments.

Action Steps for Your Body

1. MOVE-ing

2. EAT-ing

Attitude Focus for Your Brains and Bliss

1. THINK-ing

2. FEEL-ing

Take a minute to think about your past successes and write them down.

Are there any common themes in this list? What factors contributed most to your success? Use these insights as we break down these goals into smaller, more manageable segments in the next chapter.

If you find you have a mental block or can't get past these steps, I suggest you put this book down and go for a walk to clear your head. If you are still having trouble, then just keep going and come back here as you clarify your goals.

Finally, THRIVE-ing is more than just fulfilling goals. Move away now from your left-sided, list-making part of your brain and use your creative right brain to think about what THRIVE-ing feels like. What will it look like? Imagine it.

▶ WHAT I HOPE YOU WILL ACHIEVE

I have loved writing this book because my *Guide to THRIVE* is not about exercise or diet or stress management. It is about living the life you envisioned, knowing who you are and what you want to be. Sure, the tools I teach you are practical, and large segments of the book are spent learning how to care for your body, but in doing so you are caring for your brain and your mind. In the following chapters I hope you will notice yourself—begin listening to your mind, understanding your passions and motivations, and figuring out what you really want in life. Remember what the Pizza Man taught me—as soon as you figure out what you really want out of life, everything else will fall into place.

I hope you will take back control of your body. Only 30 percent of how you age is predetermined by your genetics. This means that 70 percent of your future is in your control and is determined by the lifestyle choices you make. It's time to stop blaming our mothers and take Action.

I hope you will gain confidence in the supermarket, at the table, or in the restaurant. Food is not the enemy…it is our fuel, and it is powerful.

I hope you will have the joy of renewing your brain. Intense physical exercise can make you sharper, no matter what your age. As a 44-year-old woman, I don't want to simply have 18 years of education and life experience repeated 2½ times.

Finally, I hope that in this process you will renew your mind and have a new passion for the future. You have the tools to have it all.

This is the year you THRIVE.

②

THRIVE

Months 1 and 2

"We are what we repeatedly do. Excellence, then, is not an act, but a habit."

—Aristotle

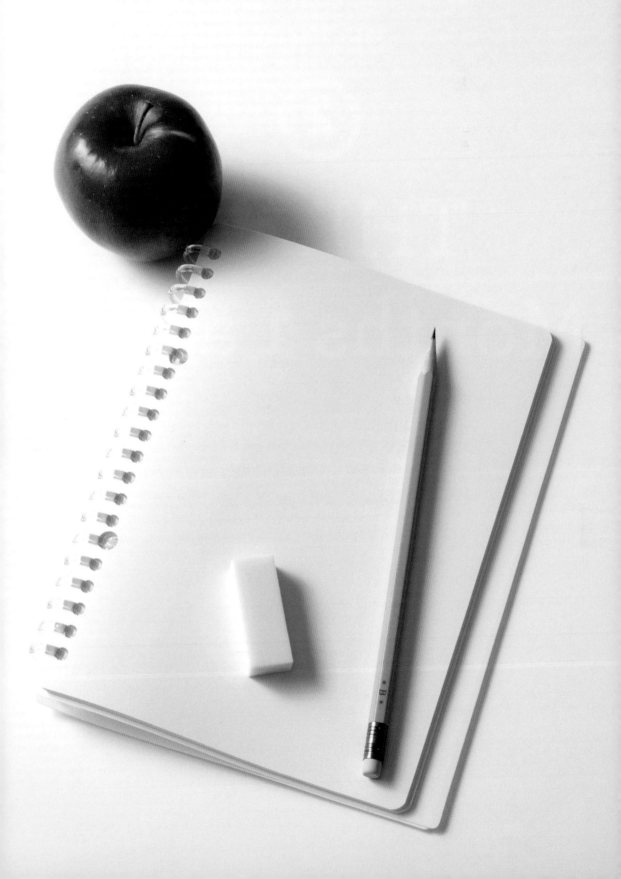

CHAPTER 5

What Does a Vision of THRIVE-ing Look Like to You?

"The only limit to our realization of tomorrow will be our doubts of today. Let us move forward with strong and active faith."
—**Franklin D. Roosevelt**

To thrive is to make "steady progress, flourishing, to grow vigorously," according to Webster. That sounds great. It's a place we would all like to be, but it is very nonspecific. What does THRIVE-ing feel like to you? Will you know it when you are there? The reason I asked you to imagine the Vision you created and to envision what THRIVE-ing would look like is that it is more than just checking off goals. It is an overall sense of well-being in the physical, mental, and emotional parts of life.

If it is hard to picture exactly what THRIVE-ing looks like, you can do a reverse thought. There is a phenomenon in children and the elderly termed "Failure to Thrive." It is a conglomeration of physical, mental, and emotional factors leading to difficulty maintaining healthy weight, lack of motivation, poor social interaction, and flat affect. The kids just don't have that spark of life—physically, mentally, or emotionally. It's as if the baby or elder has little interest in themselves or their surroundings. They are just surviving. Now think of a THRIVE-ing child. Rosy, energetic, interactive, exploring life, learning new lessons, and sprouting new neurons every minute. Now in the same way, make the contrast as you think about what THRIVE-ing means to you.

To solidify your right-brain picture of THRIVE-ing, draw it or engage your left-brain by writing it down.

Refresh and refine your six-month goals and write them below. Each should contain an element of what you are going to accomplish, how you will accomplish it, and how you will measure success. See my goals for you in the sidebar as examples.

Body: MOVE-ing

Body: EAT-ing

Attitude focus for your Brains and Bliss:

Brains: THINK-ing

Bliss: FEEL-ing

MY GOALS FOR MONTHS 1–2

» MOVE: THRIVE-ers will engage their bodies and engage their brains by learning to make the first MOVE with 25 TBT exercises and developing a daily habit of MOVE-ing.

» EAT: THRIVE-ers will know themselves by keeping a food journal, learning the 500 rule, making simple food substitutions to simplify eating, and choosing more healthy foods.

» THINK: THRIVE-ers will stimulate their brains to learn new information by MOVE-ing, and they will free up brain space with stress-reduction methods for simplifying their lives.

» FEEL: THRIVE-ers will identify what makes them happy, create a joy and thankfulness list, and fortify important relationships.

WHAT DOES A VISION OF THRIVE-ING LOOK LIKE TO YOU?

Now, what can you accomplish in eight weeks? If you are just starting out, bite off a small chunk and start simple. For instance: "I will invest time to MOVE three days per week for the first four weeks."

Action Steps for Your Body

MOVE-ing:

EAT-ing:

Attitude Focus for Your Brains and Bliss

THINK-ing:

FEEL-ing:

Setting small, manageable goals puts us in a position to succeed. Pile a few successes in front of one another, and not only have we paved the way to our goals, but succeeding becomes a habit, our mode of operation. Now let's look forward and make a MOVE.

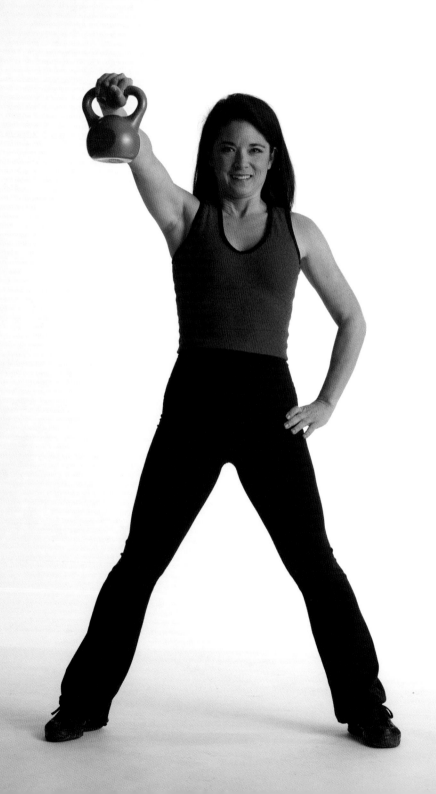

CHAPTER 6

Make the First MOVE

"The critical ingredient is getting off your butt and doing something. It's as simple as that. A lot of people have ideas, but there are few who decide to do something about them now. Not tomorrow. Not next week. But today. The true entrepreneur is a doer, not a dreamer."

—Nolan Bushnell

Everywhere you look these days there are experts, celebrities, and the gal next door telling you how to get the flattest belly, the best butt ever, or the perfect body. It can be confusing and overwhelming. MOVE-ing, however, doesn't have to be rocket science. Our bodies have an amazing capacity to adapt and prosper no matter how we move them. It is most important to make the first move!

▶ **MAKE A MOVE** *and Save Your Life*

Making a MOVE is about more than reaching the perfect dress size or looking good at your high school reunion. We are designed to MOVE. We have two strong legs and a core meant to keep us on the go our entire lives. As an orthopaedic surgeon, my passion for saving mobility has led me to the realization that by saving mobility we are actually saving lives. Did you know that there are 33 chronic diseases whose severity is diminished by a mere 30 minutes of exercise per day? Collectively these diseases are called "Sedentary Death Syndrome" and lead to more than 250,000 deaths per year. Invest 30 minutes in saving your life today. You are worth it!

Just 30 minutes of brisk aerobic exercise per day is amazing medicine. If you do it, you'll have a:

✓ **40 percent lower risk of developing diabetes. Exercise can also decrease a diabetic's risk of dying from heart disease by 40 to 50 percent.**

✓ **40 percent decrease in the risk of colorectal cancer and decrease in the risk of dying from prostate cancer by 50 percent.**

✓ **60 percent lower risk of developing breast and ovarian cancer, as exercise effectively lowers levels of two ovarian hormones, estradiol and progesterone. Brisk exercise is the only factor known to decrease the risk of breast cancer recurrence.**

✓ **1.5 x lower chance of suffering from depression than a sedentary person. Healthy, active bodies can keep your mind healthy, too.**

✓ **41 percent less erectile dysfunction than men who sit on the couch. What is good for the heart muscle is good for your penis.**

For many of my patients, making the first move means simply going for a brisk walk after dinner, throwing a few Total Body THRIVE (TBT) exercises into each TV commercial break, or taking the pile of clothes and clutter off of your treadmill and turning it on. It sounds easy, and it is.

Whether you are MOVE-ing for the first time in years or you are a lifelong exerciser, this chapter is designed to build a menu of Total Body THRIVE (TBT) exercises that maximize performance and minimize injury in every part of your body. Every two weeks I will teach you a short set of new exercises, and by Week 8 you will know 25 ways to strengthen and tone your whole body. We progress from doing sets of single exercises in Weeks 1-4 to building short but intense exercise circuits in Weeks 5-8.

▶ **THRIVE** *Principles*

1. Short, intense Total Body Workout
2. USE gravity
3. Ground reactive forces
4. Confuse our muscles

With short workouts you are more likely to stick with the program. This makes exercising fun and intense. I call this fun, intense circuit training Powerplay.

Our bodies are amazing adaptation machines, and a little means a lot. Short intense total body sessions not only go a long way toward building a THRIVE-ing body but also serve as the stimulus for making growth factors to feed our brains and revive our minds (Bliss). We get Body, Brains, and Bliss!

The TBT exercises can be performed anywhere—from your living room to the gym—and do not require heavy equipment. I believe that the most effective exercise mimics life and am therefore not a huge advocate for weight machines. In life, our muscle groups work in coordination with each other. They push and pull against gravity while being pushed upon by the ground reactive force. Machines artificially work one muscle group at a time without the added benefits of gravity.

For instance, when you go up and down stairs, climb hills, and squat down, your knees are under tremendous pressure. Weak or imbalanced leg and core muscles are not strong enough to stabilize your kneecaps, and this leads to knee pain. Strengthening your quads with a traditional leg press machine takes gravity out of the picture and works your quads in only one direction. I teach my patients total body exercises, such as wall squats, to regain real-life strength in the butt, core, and quads.

Finally, for the greatest benefit, we must not only MOVE intensely in the functional way our bodies live, but we must also confuse our muscles. Our 650 muscles are built for efficiency. With repetition they not only get stronger but adapt to use the least amount of energy for any given motion. That is why doing the same exercise becomes easy after a while. The TBT exercise circuits are designed to keep your muscles guessing. They work in a new way every few weeks and never get a chance to rest on their laurels. Your muscles just keep THRIVE-ing.

▶ WEEKS 1–8: *Getting Your MOVE On*

The secret to getting started is breaking down big tasks to small, manageable pieces. The following pages teach you the first TBT exercises and suggest a weekly schedule. You must make this timing work for you. It doesn't matter which days you choose for TBT versus aerobic exercise as long as you make the time. When you are able, you can actually stack the TBT and aerobic portions in the same day. Your goal is 2–3 days per week of TBT exercises and 3–5 days per week of aerobic exercise. Each workout is preceded by a dynamic warm-up to get your blood pumping, warm up your muscles, and put you in the best frame of mind. At the end of this chapter are THRIVE homework pages to help you track your progress and plan your rewards.

Sample Schedule

	Mon	Tues	Wed	Thurs	Fri	Sat	Sun	Comments
Weeks 1-4	DW/TBT	DW/ A	DW/ TBT	DW/ A	rest	DW/ TBT/A	rest	DW/daily A/ 3-5 times / wk TBT1/2-3 times/wk
Weeks 5-6	DW/ TBTC1	DW/ A	DW/ TBTC1	DW/ A	rest	DW/ TBTC1/ A	rest	TBTC1- 45 sec per exercise/ 15 sec rest
Weeks 7-8	DW/ TBTC2	DW/ A	DW/ TBTC2	DW/ A	rest	DW/ TBTC2/ A	rest	TBTC2- 45 sec per exercise/ 15 sec rest

DW = dynamic warm-up, TBT= Total Body THRIVE exercises, A = aerobic,
TBTC 1 = Total Body THRIVE circuit #1, TBTC 2 = total body THRIVE circuit #2

▶ EXERCISE TIPS

Engage Your Core

The "core" is hot these days. Everyone is talking about it—and with good reason. Our power to do everything from sit up in bed, walk to our next meeting, balance upright without falling down, and blast through our next workout comes from this muscle group. These muscles even protect us from the menace of low back pain. It is no wonder that this central real estate houses some of our body's biggest muscles.

But what and where exactly is the core? Just as its name implies, the core is right in the middle of our bodies. These three sheets of muscle wrap like a belt around the central part of our bodies and connect our spine to our belly. These oblique muscles are responsible for all the bending, twisting, pulling, pushing, and spine support that goes into every minute activity. Many people mistake the "six pack," which graces the pages of so many fitness magazines, as the goal. Instead, it is the muscles that twist around the sides of our body to form the natural weight belt that powers our movement.

To engage your core, simply place both hands on the sides of your body at the level of your navel and bear down like someone was about to punch you in the stomach. You should feel the oblique sheets of muscle harden. This is the feeling you want prior to any exercise.

Breathe

You have been doing this since before you can remember, yet many people hold their breath while they are exercising or breathe so inefficiently they add more work to their workout. Simply breathe in through your nose and out through your mouth in a long, controlled flow. When you are exerting energy, such as pushing, pulling, or lifting, you exhale. When you are relaxing the move or lowering the weight, you inhale.

Shoulders Over Elbows

By design, our shoulders were made to allow extreme motion in multiple directions. They were not designed for bearing weight. Many of our exercises, however, from the simple push-up to the plank, require we hold up our weight with our shoulders and upper bodies. To prevent shoulder injury and to get the most out of your exercise, always make sure your shoulders are lined up directly over your elbows and hands.

Knees Over Ankles

Our poor knees are stuck in the middle. Hip, ankle, leg, and butt weakness can all manifest as knee pain. To protect these innocent bystanders from further stress during the TBT exercises, make sure your knee is always positioned directly above your ankle. This minimizes the stress placed across the front of your kneecap and puts your leg in a more mechanically stable position. Check your look in the mirror if you need to.

▶ TOTAL BODY THRIVE (TBT)
Exercise Summary

In the sample schedule, you see a workout suggestion for each day of the week for Weeks 1–8. The daily regimen consists of combinations of workouts such as DW: Dynamic Warm-Ups and TBTC: Total Body THRIVE Circuits. The following section gives an overview of the exercises in each workout and finally I demonstrate them. Refer to the Homework section for weekly workout charts.

Dynamic Warm-Up

To start your Powerplay and minimize injury, warm up dynamically before every TBT and aerobic workout. These exercises activate your muscles, loosen your joints, get your blood pumping, and signal your brain to get into an exercise frame of mind.

- ✓ **Hip rotations**
- ✓ **Foam roller**
- ✓ **Activator**
- ✓ **High knee-to-chest lunge**

TBT Weeks 1–4:

Weeks 1–2 begin by learning five total body exercises performed 2–3 times per week. In Weeks 3 and 4 you learn a new set of five total body exercises that build on Weeks 1–2. These are all performed as simple reps or sets. Refer to the weekly homework charts starting on page 92.

Total Body Focus	Weeks 1-2	Weeks 3-4
Core	Plank	Side plank
Buttocks	Monster walk	Hip raises
Quads	Prisoner squat	Spilt squat
Chest/back	Push-ups	W.I. on ball
Shoulders	Scaption/shrug	Rotator cuff

TBT Circuit 1 (TBTC1) Weeks 5–6:

Now that you know the first 10 exercises, it's time to throw your muscles a curve ball. On TBT days during Weeks 5 and 6, combine the ten exercises you learned into a continuous circuit. Perform each exercise for 45 seconds with 15 seconds of rest in between. One TBT circuit should take you approximately 10 minutes to complete. TBT circuits add intensity to the exercises you already know and will keep your heart rate up for the duration. When you are finished with one circuit, let's see how F.A.R. you can go and try another.

TBT Circuit 2 (TBTC2) Weeks 7–8:

At this point your body has been THRIVE-ing for six weeks and is used to working for you, building up a sweat, and getting stronger. Now throw your muscles another curveball by learning a new 10-exercise circuit. Again, perform each exercise for 45 seconds with 15 seconds of rest in between.

Total Body Focus		
Core	Mountain climber	Oblique chop
Buttocks	Half squat with kettle bell	Kettle bell swing
Quads	Balance reach (3 dir.)	Airplane
Chest/Back	Curl to lunge to press	Chair dip
Shoulders	Back row	T.Y. on ball

Aerobic Exercise

We need to get your heart rate up for 20–30 intense minutes 3–5 times per week. Remember this is Powerplay. You are THRIVE-ing your entire body into great shape *and* having fun. There are a multitude of ways to MOVE aerobically, and you should experiment to find the method that works for you. The aerobic part of your week doesn't have to be the same every day, either. Remember, MOVE-ing should be intense and fun. This is how adults play!

If you are just starting out with aerobic exercise, I suggest the walk/run method to MOVE. You have been walking and running since you were about a year old, so this is easy. The only difference now is that we are building up stamina. I teach my patients and exercisers the "perceived effort" plan to add intensity to and eliminate any chance of boredom.

You can determine your "effort" by monitoring your heart rate with a heart-rate monitor, taking your pulse, or simply by listening to your body work.

   1. 5-minute walking warm-up, or use the TBT dynamic warm-up.

   2. 2-minute run at 90 percent maximum effort

   3. 2-minute walk/jog at 65 percent maximum effort

   4. 2-minute run at 90 percent maximum effort

   5. 2-minute walk/jog at 65 percent maximum effort

   6. 2-minute run at 90 percent maximum effort

   7. 2-minute walk/jog at 65 percent maximum effort

   8. 5-minute walk recovery

   ✓ Depending on your speed, you should be able to cover between
       1–1.5 miles with this 17-minute pattern. Just repeat steps
       2–7 until you cover the distance or time you desire.

✓ As you THRIVE and this schedule is not a challenge, or you need to cover more distance in less time, make the runs three minutes and the walks 1 minute.

✓ When this schedule is not a challenge, or you need to cover more distance in less time, make the runs four minutes and the walks two minutes.

✓ At the end of the program, you should be able to run for five minutes at a time with a 1–2 minute walk/jog in between as necessary.

✓ But what if you can't stand to run? Never fear. The perceived effort/time method works for any means of aerobic activity, including straight running, spinning, the treadmill, elliptical machine, rowing, and even jumping rope.

▶ BURN THE BIG 500

Below are the big ten aerobic exercises that burn approximately 500 calories per hour in a 130-pound woman.

1. Rowing (vigorous effort)	502
2. Running 5.2 mph (11.5 minute mile)	531
3. Ice skating 9 mph	531
4. Kickboxing	590
5. Rock climbing (ascending)	649
6. Cross-country skiing (vigorous effort)	531
7. Swimming laps freestyle (vigorous effort)	590
8. Bicycling 14–15.9 mph (vigorous effort)	590
9. Walking up stairs	472
10. Running up stairs	885

▶ DYNAMIC WARM-UP: *Perform Daily Prior to TBT or Aerobic Exercise*

✓ **Hip rotations**

✓ **Foam roller**

✓ **Activator**

✓ **High knee-to-chest lunge**

Hip Rotations: Hip Joint, Core, Butt, Balance Builder

1. Begin with hands on hips and feet together. Engage your core.

2. Raise one leg up in front of the body at the hip and rotate it out to the side in a circle, then lower it.

3. Reverse by raising the leg up to the side of the body at the hip and rotating it to the front.

4. Repeat ten times and switch to the opposite leg.

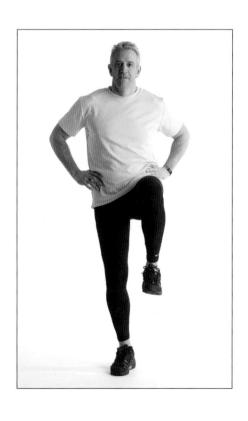
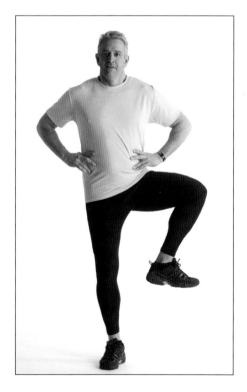

Foam Roller: ITB, Buttocks, Quads, Hamstrings, Calves

1. Place the roller of foam directly under the muscle group to be stretched.

2. Place your full body weight on the roller. This may be uncomfortable, but that is all right.

3. Pull your body back and forth slowly over the roller using your upper body. Imagine your are the rolling pin and the roller is the dough.

4. Roll five times over each muscle group. Repeat on opposite side.

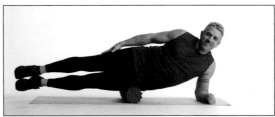

IT Band

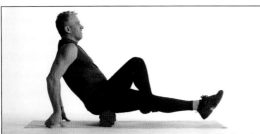

Buttocks

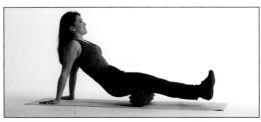

Hamstrings

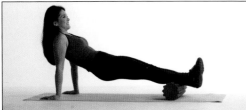

Calves

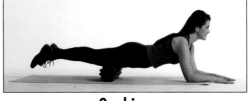

Quadriceps

Activator: Ankles, Knees, Hips, Hamstrings, Butt

1. Begin in a push-up position with your weight on your hands and toes.

2. Engage your core and keep your back flat from shoulders to ankles.

3. Walk your ankles toward your shoulders keeping your knees straight. Continue walking forward until the stretch in the back of your legs is uncomfortable.

4. Keep your back straight, not allowing it to arch.

5. Pause at the top. Slowly walk your hands forward with your feet still until you are back in the push-up position.

6. Perform five cycles.

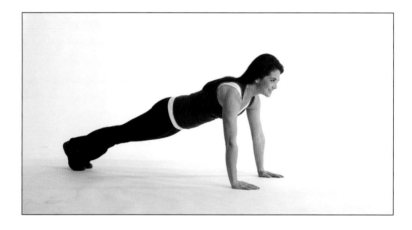

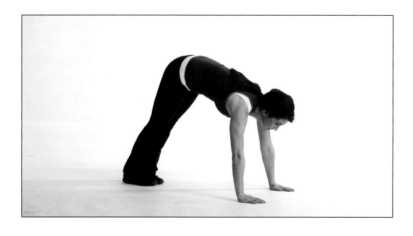

High Knee-to-Chest Lunge: Hips, Butt, Hip Flexors, Balance

1. Stand with your feet together and engage your core.

2. In a controlled manner, raise one of your knees to your chest and hold with your arms. Pause in this position to gain control of your balance. Your back should be straight and shoulders back.

3. Lunge forward on the raised leg, keeping your knee above your ankle. Keep your core engaged and your butt tucked under to maximize the hip flexor stretch portion of the lunge.

4. Perform five per side.

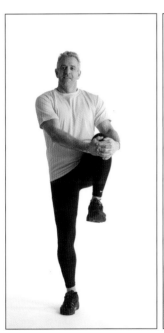
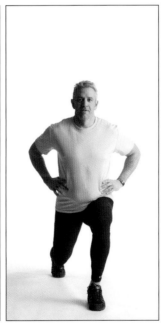
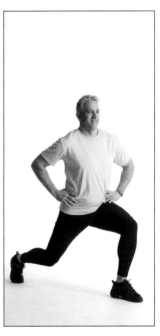

▶ TBT WEEKS 1–4 (TBT)

Total Body Focus	Weeks 1-2	Weeks 3-4
Core	Plank	Side plank
Buttocks	Monster walk	Hip raises
Quads	Prisoner squat	Split squat
Chest/back	Push-ups	W.I. on ball
Shoulders	Scaption/shrug	Rotator cuff

Plank: Core

1. Get into a push-up position but bend your elbows and place weight on your forearms instead of your hands.

2. Lower your buttocks until your back is flat and your body is in a straight line from ankles to shoulders. Engage your core by pulling your navel toward your spine and pushing down as if you were going to be punched in the gut. Make sure your butt is not sticking up or sinking down.

3. Hold for 30 seconds and work up to two minutes. Remember to breathe.

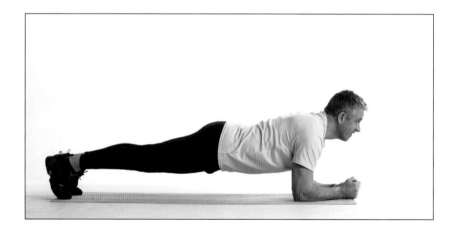

Monster Walk: Gluteus Medius

1. Place a resistance band or continuous exercise band just above your ankles.

2. Place your feet approximately shoulder-width apart with gentle tension on the band. Engage your core. Slightly bend your knees and hips.

3. Take a half step to the side with the right foot and then follow with a half step toward the right foot with the left. Maintain tension on the band at all times.

4. Take ten steps to the right and then reverse to the left. Feel the burn in the top of your buttocks.

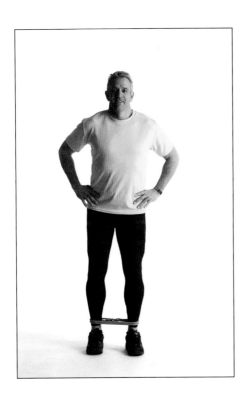
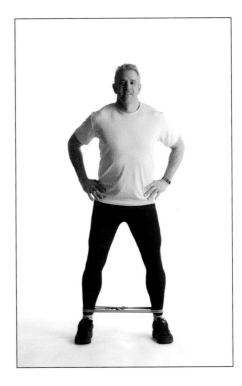

Prisoner Squat: Quads, Core, Butt, Legs

1. Engage your core and stand with your feet shoulder-width apart.

2. Hold your arms straight out in front of your shoulders.

3. Lower your body until your butt is parallel to your knees by pushing your butt back and bending your knees. Try to keep your knees above your ankles.

4. Keep your back flat and chest upright.

5. Keep your weight on your heels, not your toes.

6. Perform two sets of 10.

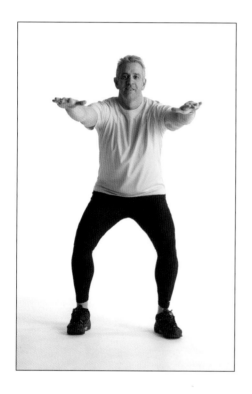
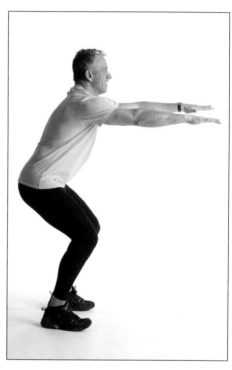

Push-Ups: Chest, Biceps, Triceps, Core

1. Get down on your hands and toes with your hands a little wider than your shoulders. Legs are straight, core is engaged, and butt is tight. Your body is a straight line from shoulders to toes.

2. Lower your body by bending your elbows until your chest is level with your elbows. (Going all the way to the floor puts excessive pressure on the front of the shoulders.)

3. Pause at the bottom and push back up to the starting position.

4. Do not let your butt sag during the push-up.

5. Work up to 10.

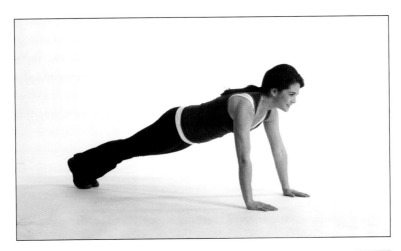

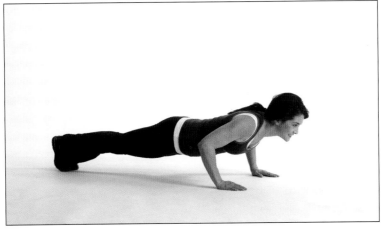

Scaption/Shrug: Shoulders

1. Stand with your feet shoulder-width apart, and engage your core.

2. Roll your shoulders back by squeezing your back muscles together and stand up straight.

3. Raise your arms in the front of your body so they form a Y.

4. Shrug your shoulders and pause in that position, then return slowly to the starting position.

5. Perform two sets of 10.

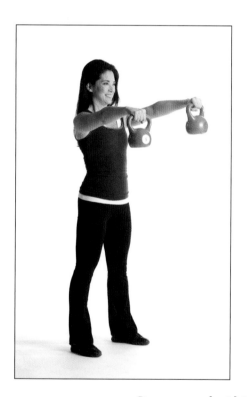 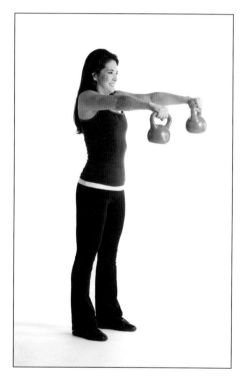

**Demonstrated with THRIVE Kettle Bells,
sold exclusively at Dick's Sporting Goods stores.**

▶ TBT WEEKS 3–4

Side Plank: Oblique Core

1. Lie on your side and raise up onto your elbow. Place your weight on your forearm and the side of your lower foot. Engage your core and squeeze your butt.

2. Raise your trunk off the floor and lower your buttocks until your body is a straight line from ankles to shoulders. Make sure your butt is not sticking up or sinking down. Your shoulder should be directly over your elbow.

3. Hold for 30 seconds and work up to two minutes. Remember to breathe.

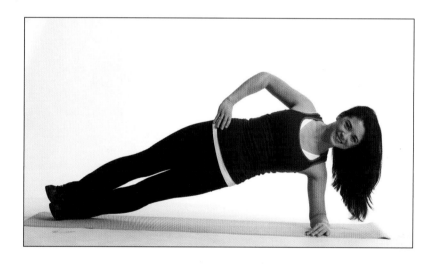

Hip Raises on Exercise Ball: Butt, Hamstrings, Core

1. Lie face up on the floor and place your lower legs on an exercise ball.

2. Engage your core and squeeze your butt.

3. Raise your hips off the floor so your body is straight from your shoulders to your knees.

4. Hold at the top for five seconds and return to starting position.

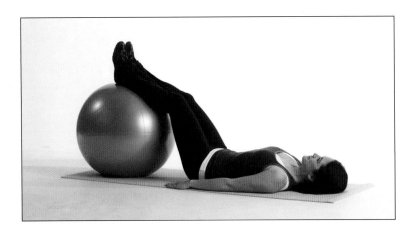

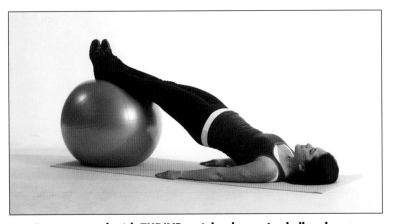

Demonstrated with THRIVE weighted exercise ball and mat, sold exclusively at Dick's Sporting Goods stores.

Split Squat: Quads, Calves, Core, Butt

1. Stand with your left foot in front of your right in a staggered stance with your front knee slightly bent and your weight on the heel of the front foot and toes of the back.

2. Engage your core and squeeze your butt.

3. Slowly lower your body until your hip is parallel to your front knee. Your front knee should be over your ankle and the back knee nearly touching the floor. Keep your torso upright.

4. Pause in this position while squeezing your butt and rotating your hips slightly forward. Push back up to starting position quickly.

5. Perform two sets of 10 on each leg.

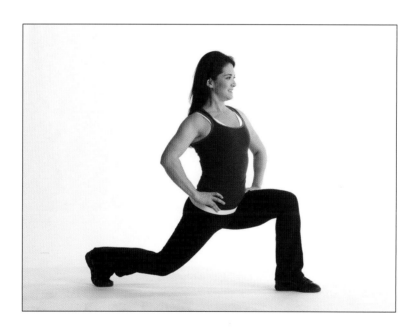

W.I. on the Exercise Ball: Shoulders, Upper Back, Core

1. Place an exercise ball under your hips and engage your core, keeping your back flat and your chest off the ball.

For W:

2. Bend your elbows to 90 degrees.

3. Rotate your elbows by squeezing your upper back muscles until your arms form a W.

4. Hold three seconds and return to starting position.

5. Perform two sets of 10.

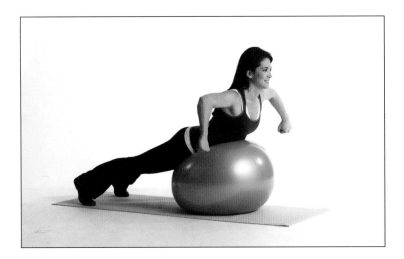

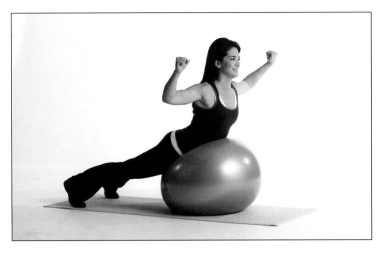

For I:

2. Extend your elbows directly down toward the floor with palms in and thumbs forward.

3. Raise your arms up until they are in line with your body by squeezing your upper back muscles.

4. Hold three seconds and return to the starting position.

5. Perform two sets of 10.

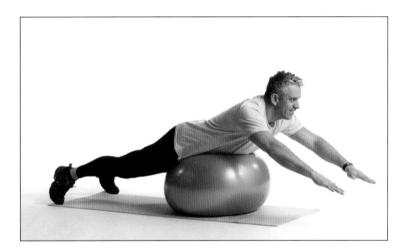

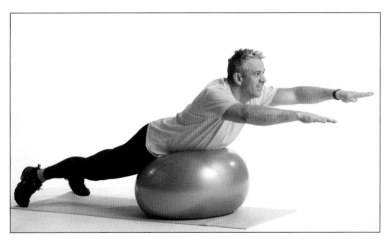

Rotator Cuff/Shoulder in Four Planes: Forward Flexion, Cross Arm Abduction, Internal and External Rotation

Forward Flexion

1. Stand with your feet shoulder-width apart. Engage your core.

2. Place one end of an exercise band under your right foot and hold the opposite end with your right hand. (This can also be performed with a hand weight.)

3. With shoulder blades squeezed together, slowly raise your arm forward in the plane of your shoulder and pause at the top before returning to the starting position.

4. One set of 10 for each arm.

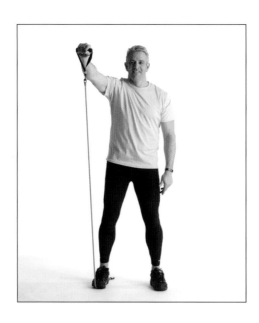

Cross Arm Abduction

1. Stand with your feet shoulder-width apart. Engage your core.

2. Place the end of the band under your left foot, and keep the other end in your right hand.

3. With shoulder blades squeezed together, raise your arm across your body in a V motion until it is level with your shoulder.

4. Pause at the top before returning to the starting position.

5. One set of 10 for each arm.

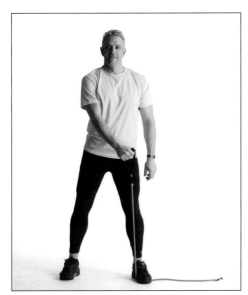 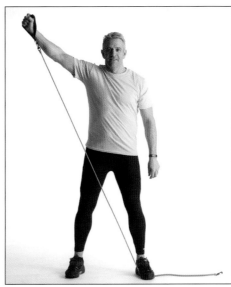

External Rotation

1. Place one end of the band around a sturdy object and stand with your left side toward the object.

2. Place the other end of the band in your right hand.

3. Keep your elbow next to your body and pull the band away from your body.

4. Pause at maximal external rotation before returning to starting position.

5. One set of 10 on each side.

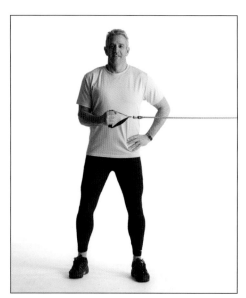
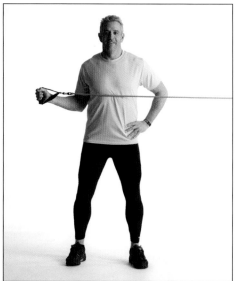

Internal rotation

1. Place one end of the band around a sturdy object and stand with your right side toward the object.

2. Place the other end of the band in your right hand.

3. With your elbow next to your body, pull the band across your body.

4. Pause at maximal internal rotation before returning to the starting position.

5. One set of 10 on each side.

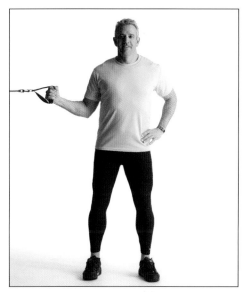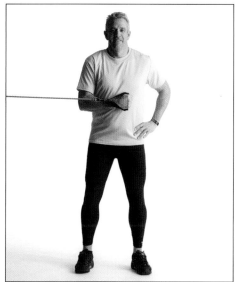

▶ TBT WEEK 5–6 CIRCUIT (TBTC1)

During weeks 5 and 6, combine the 10 exercises you learned in Weeks 1–4 in circuit. Powerplay 45 seconds for each exercise with 15 seconds of rest in between.

▶ TBT WEEK 7–8 CIRCUIT (TBTC2)

Powerplay 45 seconds for each exercise with 15 seconds of rest in between.

Total Body Circuit		
Core	Mountain climber	Oblique chop
Buttocks	Half squat with kettle bell	Kettle bell swing
Quads	Balance reach- 3 dir.	Airplane
Chest/back	Curl to lunge to press	Chair dip
Shoulders	Back row	T.Y. on ball

Mountain Climber: Core Stability for Spine Support, Abdominal Strength

1. Engage your core and assume a push-up position with your arms straight and your body forming a straight line from shoulders to ankles.

2. Lift your right foot off the floor and bring your knee toward the chest as far as you can. Keep your back straight.

3. Return to the starting position and switch legs.

4. Alternate back and forth for 45 seconds.

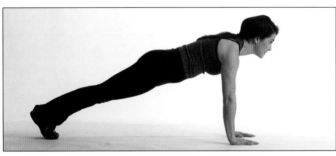

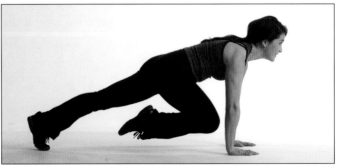

Half Squat with Kettle Bell: Butt, Quads, Core Stability, Upper Back

1. Start in the prisoner squat position with your back flat and knees over your toes. Hold the kettle bell with both hands in front of you on the ground.

2. Engage your core.

3. Thrust up to a standing position using your core and butt, and bring the kettle bell up to chest level while squeezing your shoulder blades together.

4. Pause at the top and return to the starting position.

5. Perform for 45 seconds.

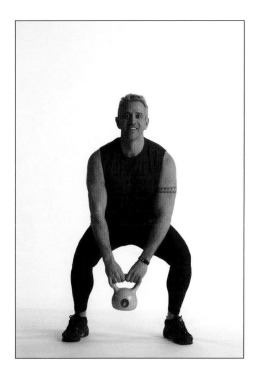
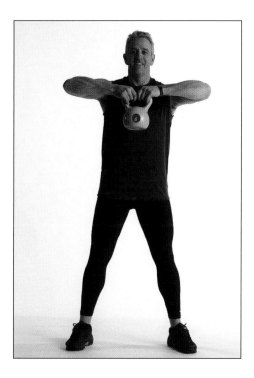

Balance Reach: Quads, Core, Balance

1. Engage your core and stand with feet together and hands on hips. Imagine you are standing in the center of a clock.

2. Reach forward with your right toe toward 12:00 while slightly bending your left knee. Keep your hips level and back straight. Pause and return to standing. Repeat to 12:00 ten times.

3. Repeat balance reach to 3:00 to the side and 6:00 to the back with the right leg.

4. Switch sides and repeat balance reach sequence with the left leg.

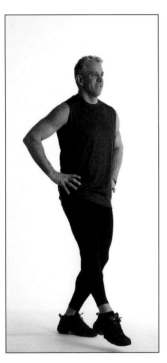 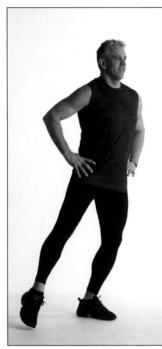 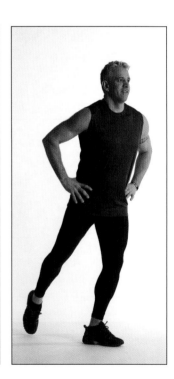

Curl to Lunge to Press: Chest, Back, Core, Butt

1. Hold a pair of mini toning balls at arms' length at your sides with your feet shoulder-width apart. Engage your core.

2. Lunge forward with your left leg. Keep your knee directly over your foot. The back knee does not touch the floor. Curl the balls as you lunge with palms facing in.

3. While in a lunge, press the balls directly overhead.

4. Push off the front leg and return to the starting position.

5. Repeat with the right leg.

6. Perform for 45 seconds.

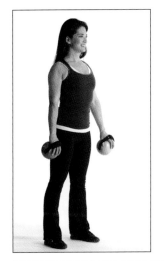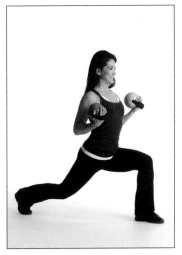
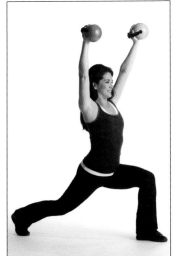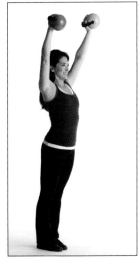

**Demonstrated using the THRIVE toning balls,
sold exclusively at Dick's Sporting Goods stores.**

Back Row: Shoulders, Upper Back

1. Loop or attach the center of a resistance band around a stable object (door, friend).

2. Hold the ends and stand with your feet shoulder-width apart. Engage your core.

3. Keep your body rigid and squeeze your shoulder blades together as you bring the bands toward your chest at a 90-degree angle.

4. Pause and return to the starting position.

5. Perform for 45 seconds.

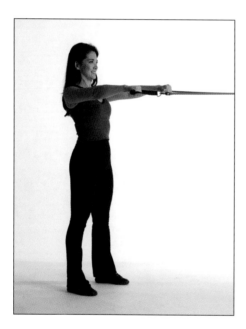 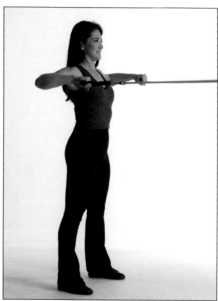

Oblique Chop: Oblique Core

1. Stand with your feet shoulder-width apart, back straight, and core engaged.

2. Hold a kettle bell or free weight in both hands next to the right shoulder. (The oblique chop can also be performed without weights.)

3. Bring the kettle bell across the front of your body to the outside of your left knee in a controlled manner by contracting your left oblique muscles.

4. Pause in this position, bring the kettle bell up to the left shoulder in a standing position, and repeat to the right knee.

5. Perform for 45 seconds.

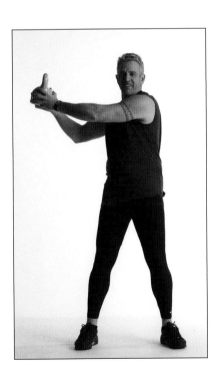 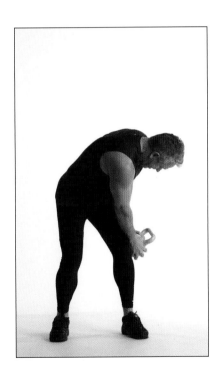

Kettle Bell Swing: Hamstrings, Butt, Core, Quads, Shoulders

1. Hold a kettle bell in your right hand at waist level at arms' length. Place your feet slightly wider than shoulder-width apart.

2. Lower into a half squat with hips pushed back and bent 60 degrees to the floor.

3. Swing the kettle bell between your legs, keeping your arm straight.

4. Thrust your hips forward, squeezing your butt together and allowing your knees to straighten to a standing position while you swing the kettle bell up to chest level.

5. Return to a squat position as you swing the kettle bell down between your legs.

6. Perform for 45 seconds.

The power of this exercise comes from your core, legs, and butt. The kettle bell swings forward from the momentum of the thrust and is not lifted with the shoulders.

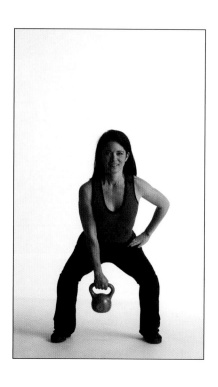
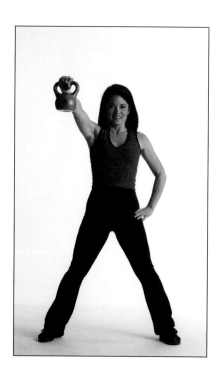

Airplane: Quads, Core, Balance

1. Stand with feet together, core engaged, and arms extended to the side at shoulder height.

2. Bend the left knee slightly and bend forward at the hips in a controlled manner with the right leg extended behind your body until your shoulders, back, and ankle form a straight line.

3. Hold in this position for five seconds to control balance with your core and return to the starting position.

4. Perform for 45 seconds.

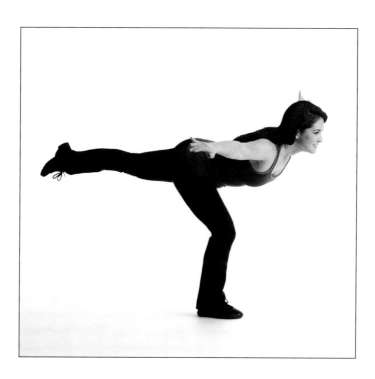

Chair Dip: Triceps, Upper Back

1. Sit on the edge of a sturdy chair and place your hands beside your hips on the chair.

2. Slide forward until your weight is on your hands and your elbows are facing back.

3. Continue lowering your body in a dip, slowly counting 1-2-3 down and 1-2-3 up.

4. Perform for 45 seconds.

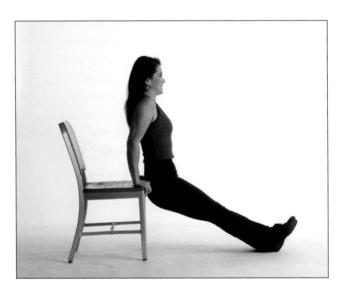

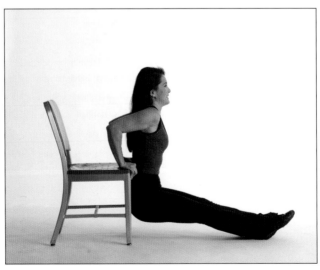

T.Y. on the Exercise Ball: Shoulders, Upper Back, Core

1. Place an exercise ball under your hips and engage your core, keeping your back flat and your chest off the ball.

For the T:

2. Arms should be in front of the ball with palms forward and thumbs out.

3. Raise your arms out to the sides with thumbs up. Keep your back flat. Your body forms a T. Hold three seconds and return to the starting position

4. Perform for 45 seconds.

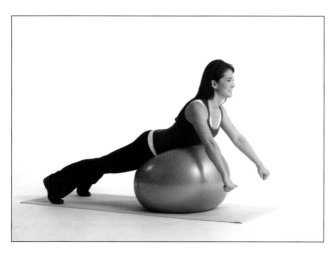

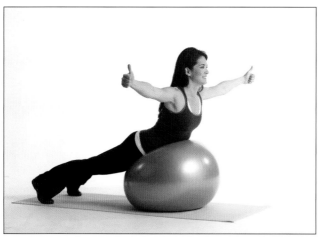

For the Y:

2. Arms should be in front of the ball with palms in and thumbs up.

3. Raise your arms in front of your body with your thumbs out 30 degrees from your shoulders. Your body forms a "Y." Hold three seconds and return to starting position.

4. Perform for 45 seconds.

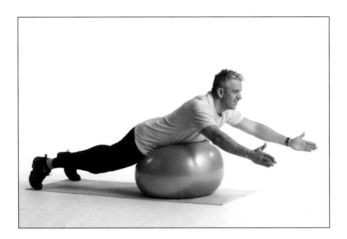

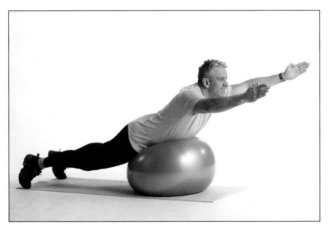

▶ LOCATION, LOCATION, LOCATION

So what is the big deal about accumulating a little fat here and there as we age? It's natural, right? The fact is that while our body composition does change as we get older, it is important to keep fat accumulation in check. Fat is not just hanging around innocently. It is a metabolically active organ producing hormones and chemicals that negatively affect our body's function and can make disease worse. Fat produces hormones that cause high blood sugar (resistin), high blood pressure (angiotensinogen), inflammation, and infiltrates that clog every tissue from blood vessels to muscles and tendons.

What we know about fat is that it is all about location, location, location! It matters where it lands. Seventy percent of how we age is due to the good or bad lifestyle choices we make, while only 30 percent can be blamed on genetics. Fat deposition is genetically determined. If you carry fat around your middle, like an apple, you are more likely to develop health problems than people who carry weight around their hips like pears. This is true even if your weight is within normal range. Apple-shaped people spend more money on health care and medication and are most at risk for developing diabetes, high cholesterol, metabolic syndrome, and all the co-morbid consequences of these diseases. These dire facts point to my urgency in teaching you to accumulate muscle and minimize fat. It is why I am convinced that saving mobility ultimately leads to saving lives.

How do you know if you are at risk? Get out your tape measure. Measure the widest part of your waist and the widest part of your hips. A waist measurement of greater than 40" for women and greater than 36" for men puts you in the highest risk category for metabolic syndrome and chronic disease. Now compare your waist-to-hip ratio. Divide your waist measurement by your hip measurement. The safest ratio for your health is less than 0.8. As your waist/hip ratio climbs to 1.0 or more, your risk of heart disease, stroke, and many other of the diseases in "sedentary death syndrome" rises several hundred percent.

Now before you read another page, get up and get going on a TBT circuit. Let's build some life-saving muscle.

▶ **TAKING ACTION** *in What You EAT*

Playing the Numbers

Many people are interested in nutrition because they want to lose weight. Good nutrition and weight loss, although related, are *not* the same thing. Nutrition is a complex subject that encompasses not only what foods our bodies need to thrive but in what quantities and at what times. Weight loss, on the other hand, is a simple numbers game.

As with exercise, it is easy to become overwhelmed by the sheer volume of advice on the who, what, when, and where of eating. It seems like every expert has different ideas. Sometimes we see side-by-side reports of carbs being good or bad, what kinds of fats we really do need, or the next miracle food. I'm sure you know what I mean.

For this reason, during months 1 and 2, I'm going to guide you to THRIVE by becoming more conscious of what you are eating and focusing on the numbers. In other words, how much you are eating, aka portion control. This is certainly not the end of the story, but it is a simple way to start. In later chapters, we will address nutrition more completely and EAT-ing to THRIVE.

First, let's learn the 500 rule. To lose a pound of fat, you must burn off 3,500 calories. To break it down into manageable chunks, this means burning off 500 calories more per day than you take in. Do this seven days in a row and you will lose one pound. The 500 rule makes weight management simple.

The 500 rule works by decreasing energy intake (food) or increasing energy output (exercise) or a combination of both. For instance, when I was trying to lose the final 10 pounds after I had my daughter, I used the 500 rule. I simply switched my daily morning coffee drink with all the pumps, milk, and fixings, with a simple cup of joe. I didn't change anything else about the way I ate initially. This simple change removed about 350 calories per day from my intake. I then made a more concentrated effort to burn 300–500 calories by exercising. In a couple of weeks, I was back to my normal weight. My patients make significant changes in their weight by eating only half of their normal portions at lunch and dinner. Initially they didn't sacrifice the foods they loved. They just enjoyed half the amount.

What if you are one of the people who say to me, "I already don't eat very much." It may be true. For you, the intense circuit-type exercise in the MOVE section will go a long way to ramp up your metabolism and build muscle. Muscle itself burns more calories in its daily work than fat, so the more of it you have, the more efficient you are at burning calories.

I suspect, however, that calories may be sneaking into your body when you are not watching. A good way to take control of your intake is to find out what you really do EAT everyday. It is easy for extra calories to sneak in when we are not consciously keeping track. For instance, this morning I took my little daughter to ballet. Before we left I made oatmeal. She ate five bites, and I ate the rest with two cups of coffee. An hour and a half later, after class, she was hungry again, so for a treat I took her to a cafe and we ordered scrambled eggs, potatoes, Canadian bacon, and milk. Again, she ate five bites and, you guessed it, I ate the rest. Today my extra calories snuck into my body off my child's plate. I tell you my side of the story because I understand how losing track happens. Even though fitness and mobility are what I talk about all the time, not recognizing ourselves in the mirror happens gradually because we are not paying attention. I get that.

In the next two weeks, I want you to pay attention and take Action in what you EAT by consciously writing down everything. I want it all—what you eat, drink, snack, and sneak from the minute you wake up until the minute you go to sleep. Use the following chart as a guide. Make sure you record the time, too. If you are eating prepared food, read the label and fill in the calories and grams of protein, fat, and carbs consumed. If you have already joined the THRIVE F.A.N. Club as discussed in chapter 2, you can use the calorie tracker online. No one will see this but you, so being detailed is best. I think you will be surprised how calories sneak in.

Weeks 1–2 EAT

Time	Food	Quantity	Approx. kcal	Fat grams	Protein grams	Carbs	Fluid		

After Week 1, review your intake. Are there high-calorie foods you consistently eat? Are you a late-night snacker, or do you crave the afternoon candy bar? Do you drink a glass of juice for breakfast? Even if weight is not an issue for you, tracking what you EAT is an amazing way to get a handle on what finds its way into your body.

During Week 2, identify where you can consistently remove 500 calories of intake a day, and don't eat or drink it. Remember the 500 calories you take out may be as simple as eliminating the wine you drink with dinner, the specialty morning coffee, or the mayonnaise on your sandwich.

Out with the Bad, In with the Good

During Weeks 3 and 4, you will continue the 500 rule daily. The next easy Action in EAT-ing to THRIVE is eliminating the obvious bad choices and making simple substitutions. This not only means a lot from the calorie standpoint, but it is our first nod toward THRIVE-ing nutrition.

The first item to eliminate is easy. Do not make or eat fried foods. Period. Almost every food you commonly fry can be prepared in a tasty and lower-calorie way—yes, even french fries. I use this example because I love french fries. In my house when I want them, I will cut golden potatoes into thin slices. Then I toss them with 1 tablespoon of olive oil. I season them with salt, pepper, or herbs, and I bake them at a high temperature in the oven until they are crispy. They are wonderful and much lower in calories than the fried version.

I don't believe in food austerity or deprivation. This makes us think even more about what we are denying ourselves. I would rather you make healthy substitutions or allow yourself the intermittent bite of chocolate cake then cut out fun food all together. I'm not saying you can't eat cake. I'm just saying you can't eat the whole piece every day.

▶ EAT-ING WELL *with Fewer Calories*

You will initially crave the foods you cut, but the truth is that our bodies adapt quickly. Believe it or not, you can crave the healthy substitutions you are making. Here are a few more suggestions:

1. Eat breakfast with protein. It makes you feel full longer.
2. Don't drown your food in oil, whether it's fried or sautéed.
3. Substitute sugar with fruit or sweeteners.
    a. Cooking with brown sugar adds 547 calories per cup versus substituting a cup of applesauce with 194 calories.
4. Avoid condiments, sauces, and salad dressing.
    a. BBQ sauce has 30 calories per tablespoon, while ketchup has 14.
    b. Season with herbs rather than sauces.
    c. Salad dressing has up to 100 calories per tablespoon.
5. Cook with cooking spray rather than oil.
6. Choose the low-calorie versions of your favorite foods.
    a. Yogurt
    b. Milk
    c. Cheese
    d. Juice
    e. Turkey rather than red meat

7. Work for your dinner by eating foods that require a lot of chewing.

8. Graze on your meal instead of eating it all at one time.

9. Remove tempting high-calorie foods from your kitchen, office, and car.

10. Focus on the problem times of day, like the 3:00 PM snack time.

Other simple categories to remove or substitute include fruit juice. Full-calorie fruit juice has 50 calories per ounce, so your morning cup of orange juice can add almost 500 calories. Substitute with the lower-calorie versions in the stores, or mix half of your morning glass with water. The same goes for sports drinks. Many have 200–350 calories per bottle, and unless you are working out intensely for more than an hour, you don't need that kind of calorie support.

Another big calorie burden comes from salad dressing and sauces. Salads are wonderful high-fiber, high-vitamin, and high-mineral entrees, but they can be surprisingly high-calorie meals when you use salad dressing. Many salad dressings contain 50–100 calories per tablespoon! When was the last time you put only one tablespoon of dressing on your salad? Try doctoring up your lettuce with lemon juice or vinegar and a small amount of oil.

After fried foods, fruit juices, and salad dressing, think about lowering the empty calories of mixed drinks, low-nutrient processed foods, and those times you cook with fat and oil. (Even olive oil has 1,920 calories per cup.) If you get a handle on these six items, you can go a long way toward controlling your calorie intake and using the 500 rule. It really isn't rocket science.

At the end of the third, sixth, and eighth weeks, you should weigh yourself. Again, you can't know where you are going unless you know where you are. What you may notice at Week 6 and Week 8 is that the scale has not changed dramatically. Don't worry—just remember that muscle weighs more than fat. Also note that your clothes are fitting differently, you are more toned, and you have more energy. This is because during your eight weeks of TBT, you have gained strength, muscle, and endurance while burning fat. The numbers on the scale reflect your growth of healthy muscle.

Know Your Numbers

In addition to the 500 rule, your weight, and your waist/hip ratio, the last number you should know during your these first two months is how many calories your body uses in your everyday activities. The resting metabolic rate (RMR) is the number of calories the body requires at rest. It is important because any calorie intake above this resting metabolic rate (RMR) is stored as fat by your body.

The RMR is a good estimate for those of us without access to complex laboratory testing of oxygen consumption and carbon dioxide gas production. The basic formula for estimating RMR at rest is:

$$\text{Body weight (pound)} \times 10 = \text{RMR}$$
$$\text{or}$$
$$\text{Body weight (kilogram)} \times 22 = \text{RMR}$$

The RMR, however, is dependent on both your weight and your activity level. The more active you are, the more energy you expend and the more calories it takes to fuel you. This is why the 500 rule and any of the many and various "diet" plans work. It's not rocket science—it is simple math. They simply assist you to burn more or consume fewer calories than your body requires as maintenance. The following table summarizes the estimated energy requirements (EER) for men and women of different heights, weights, and activity levels.

Estimated Energy Requirements (EER) for Men and Women 30 Years of Age and Older

Height (m[in])	Activity Level	Weight for BMI of 18.5kg/m2 (kg[lb])	Weight for BMI of 24.99kg/m2 (kg[lb])	EER Men Kcal/day BMI 18.5	BMI 24.99	EER Women Kcal/day BMI 18.5	BMI 24.99
1.5 (59)	Sedentary	41.6 (92)	56.2(124)	1848	2080	1625	1762
	Low Active			2009	2267	1803	1956
	Active			2215	2506	2025	2198
	Very Active			2554	2898	2291	2489
1.65							
(65)	Sedentary	50.4 (111)	68 (150)	2068	2349	1816	1982
	Low Active			2254	2566	2016	2202
	Active			2490	2842	2267	2477
	Very Active			2880	3296	2567	2807
1.80							
(71)	Sedentary	59.9 (132)	81 (178)	2301	2635	2015	2211
	Low Active			2513	2884	2239	2459
	Active			2782	3200	2519	2769
	Very Active			3225	3720	2855	3141

Reproduced from the Food and Nutrition Board, Institute of Medicine, National Academies.

Example: A 30-year-old sedentary female who is 65 inches tall and weighs 150 pounds has a BMI of 24.99. Her EER is 1,982 Kcal per day.

This means a 2,000-calorie diet will actually cause her to gain or maintain her weight unless she plays the 500 rule and/or ramps up her activity.

Taking Action

This chapter is packed with activity. Your Brain is probably THRIVE-ing from the workout of reading it. Start this very minute to invest time in your Body. Although the idea of making the first MOVE and playing the numbers as you EAT is not hard, I know that stepping away from the couch or out the door for the first time in years is not easy. What is important is that you do take Action and make the first MOVE. You are worth the time you invest.

This is the year you will THRIVE.

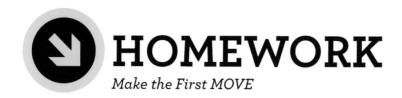

HOMEWORK

Make the First MOVE

Take Action now by MOVE-ing and EAT-ing to THRIVE. Use the following charts to track your progress and plan your rewards.

TBT Week 1–2 MOVE	Reps/time	Mon	Tues	Wed	Thurs	Fri	Sat	Sun	What worked/ What didn't/ Comments
Dynamic warm-up	**Daily**								
Hip rotations	10 per side								
Foam roller	5 per muscle group								
Activator	5 cycles								
High knee-to-chest lunge	5 per side								
TBT	**2–3 per week**								**Week 2 increase to two complete TBT**
Plank	30 sec., build to 2 minutes								
Monster walk	2 sets of 10 each leg								
Prisoner squat	2 sets of 10								
Push-ups	Work up to 10								
Scaption/ shrug	2 sets of 10								
Aerobic/ time	**3–5 per week**								
Week 1 EAT	**Track intake daily**								
Week 2 EAT	**Cut out 500 calories**								

TBT Week 3–4 MOVE	Reps/time	Mon	Tues	Wed	Thurs	Fri	Sat	Sun	What worked/ What didn't/ Comments
Dynamic warm-up	**Daily**								
Hip rotations	10 per side								
Foam roller	5 per muscle group								
Activator	5 cycles								
High knee-to-chest lunge	5 per side								
TBT	**2–3 per week**								**Week 4 increase to two complete TBT**
Side plank	30 sec., build to 2 minutes								
Hip raises	2 sets of 10								
Split squat	2 sets of 10 each leg								
W.I. on ball	2 sets of 10 each								
Rotator cuff	1 set of 10 each								
Aerobic/ time	**3–5 per week**								
Week 3 EAT	**500 rule**								**Weigh yourself**
Week 4 EAT	**Out with the bad/ in with the good**								

TBT Circuit Week 5–6 MOVE	Reps/time	Mon	Tues	Wed	Thurs	Fri	Sat	Sun	What worked/ What didn't/ Comments
Dynamic warm-up	**Daily**								
Hip rotations	10 per side								
Foam roller	5 per muscle group								
Activator	5 cycles								
High knee-to-chest lunge	5 per side								
TBT Circuit 1 45 sec. per exercise 15 sec. rest	**2 TBTC**								**If two TBTC are easy, try three**
Plank									
Monster walk									
Prisoner squat									
Push-ups									
Scaption/ shrug									
Side plank									
Hip raises									
Split squad									
W.I. on ball									
Rotator cuff									
Aerobic/ time									
Week 5 EAT	**500 rule**								
Week 6 EAT	**500 rule**								**Weigh yourself**

TBT Weeks 7–8 MOVE	Reps/time	Mon	Tues	Wed	Thurs	Fri	Sat	Sun	What worked/ What didn't/ Comments
Dynamic warm-up	**Daily**								
Hip rotations	10 per side								
Foam roller	5 cycles								
Activator	5 cycles								
High knee-to-chest lunge	5 per side								
TBT Circuit 2 45 sec. per exercise 15 sec. rest 2 TBTC	**2 TBTC**								**If two TBTC are easy, try three**
Mountain climber									
Half squat with kettle bell									
Balance reach- 3 dir.									
Mountain climber									
Half squat with kettle bell									
Oblique chop									
Kettle bell swing									
Airplane									
Chair dip									
T.Y. on ball									
Aerobic/ time	**3–5 per week**								
Week 1 EAT	**500 rule**								
Week 2 EAT	**500 rule**								**Weigh yourself**

MAKE THE FIRST MOVE

Things
TO DO

Date: _____

Priority

CHAPTER 7

Living Smarter

As a man thinketh in his heart, so is he.

—Proverbs 23:7

Y ou are making your first MOVE, and you are learning about how you EAT. Now let us clear up some space in your brain and free you to THINK and FEEL in these first two months.

When I talk to my patients about what is going on in their lives and how to make time for life-saving exercise, a common theme often arises. Women feel stressed. Most of the time it is not that they don't want to take care of themselves. But when you work, are a mother, daughter, and a community member, the demands of time, relationships, caretaking, and finances can leave women feeling out of control and with few resources for themselves.

Stress is not only a feeling but is an ancient physical defense mechanism meant to protect us from danger. It is only when stress becomes chronic that it is a problem. Here is how it works.

When you perceive danger in the form of stress from any source (a big deadline, an angry boss, financial woes, mean girls), your brain releases hormones that travel through the blood to the adrenal glands. These little stress hot spots sit on top of your kidneys and release two stress hormones that act on your entire body.

When the adrenal glands release adrenaline, you are instantly ready to fight or run. Your heart pounds to supply your muscles with blood, your bronchiol (lung) tubes dilate to bring in more oxygen, and your brain becomes more alert to assimilate and process new information. At the same time, the adrenal glands emit cortisol to release fat and glucose into the bloodstream to fuel your flight. This is a perfect system in the short term.

Trouble develops during chronic stress as cortisol levels remain high in the body. Now your body goes into survival mode and begins to store as much energy as it can for future fights. Our adrenal glands don't know that our stress is coming from our boss, not from running away from some angry boar (an angry bore, perhaps) so they continue to prepare you for the worst. This energy storage overdrive leads to metabolic disruption, muscle breakdown, high blood sugar, and belly fat storage. Chronic stress makes you fat, which just adds to your already stressed-out life.

▶ JUST BREATHE!

At any stressful point during the day, you can instantly lower your blood pressure and relax right where you are. When you breathe slowly through your nose, a gas called nitric oxide is released from your nasal passages into the bloodstream. This gas acts on the blood vessels to dilate them and lowers your blood pressure naturally. You will have moments of relaxation.

Stop reading, close your eyes, and breathe slowing through your nose for a count of ten. Exhale slowly through your mouth the same way. Repeat this 5–10 times.

Use this technique whenever you need a little breather. Under chronic stress, you take shallow breaths and may even hold them. This causes shunting of blood to the brain and makes you more alert, but it makes the kidneys less effective at filtering the salt out of your blood and explains why chronic stress can lead to high blood pressure.

Now, we are not always in control of the world around us, or the a bore at work, but we are in control of our attitudes and how we ch to respond to stressors. It is our attitude that shapes our experiences.

From the minute we are born, change—aka stress—is part of living. Some people respond to this life force in a hardy way and THRIVE on it. According to Salvatore Maddi, a UC Irvine psychologist and the father of the concept of hardiness, those people who thrive under stress maintain three attitudes of hardiness—commitment, control, and challenge.

"No matter how bad things get, if you're committed, you stay involved and give your best effort rather than pull back," Maddi said. "If you exert control and tend to perceive yourself as in charge, you try to influence the outcome of events rather than lapse into passivity. The feeling of being out of control is stressful, but planning and staying active minimizes stress. Finally, if you believe change is normal, you're more able to treat it as simply a challenge." Maddi suggested mastering this by believing in your abilities and pushing your personal envelope. "Set challenging but reachable goals that become progressively more challenging," Maddi said. "Intentionally expose yourself to things that you're afraid of." Then you should reward yourself for your success. "Give yourself credit when you do reach goals." It is the perspective that out of chaos can come many opportunities.

There are several easy strategies that go a long way toward minimizing your daily stress, simplifying your life, and de-cluttering your brain. Let's clear room to experience the joy that comes with a life full with career, family, kids, and community.

Give yourself a break. I know you want to do everything and be the best you can be in all your roles. None of us actually make goals to be mediocre. But I've come to an amazing and liberating truth in my life. I don't have to be the one doing everything for everyone in my life in order to THRIVE or have a THRIVE-ing household. The other female doctors in my group often remind ourselves that not only are we doing the surgery and patient care our male counterparts are doing every day, but we also go home and do everything their wives do in addition. I suggest you stop beating yourself up. Unless someone is going to die or your house is going to be foreclosed by you skipping your next task, give yourself permission to leave unimportant things undone, to seek out efficient solutions that free up time (order groceries online or send the babysitter to the store), to stop taking yourself so seriously since not everyone else does, and to get rid of things or superficial relationships that are weighing you down.

Change your loyalties. Just because you have shopped at the same places and used the same services for years does not mean you have to continue the same patterns if doing so adds stress to your life. Many marketers are getting smart about what today's woman needs to simplify her life. Seek out products and services that actually give you control, great customer service, ease of delivery, and ultimately, peace of mind. By doing so you are not being disloyal—you are being smart and taking care of yourself.

Stop creating more stress. Minimizing stress on a day-to-day basis means saying no, even to fun things, if they increase the burden of your life. At least once per week I say, "Let's have a party, let's have people over." In my packed life, I do not get to see the friends I care about nearly enough, and I long to see them. After an evening of friends and laughter, I am always relaxed and recharged. Putting it all together, however, adds stress. Try to live daily with an attitude of, "I choose to/not to," instead of giving up control and feeling like, "I have to." Along the same lines, it is okay not to bake the cookies for school from scratch, to say no to a new project or committee, or to blow off the tickets you bought for a concert in lieu of a quiet night at home.

▸ SAY YES CAREFULLY

When I was in medical school, I had the privilege to consult for the Pfizer Corporation where I met Dr. Mike Magee, a retired general surgeon, who then served as Pfizer's medical director. When I was finishing my fellowship in New York and was about to start my career, I revisited him to ask for advice. We talked about a lot of things, but in the end I asked him to tell me what he thought was most important as a young surgeon entering an academic career.

He explained to me that I would be asked to do a lot of different and often unrelated tasks starting out—committee work, grant writing, special projects, etc.—and that if I was not careful, these tasks could add up to a pile of projects without a unifying thread.

His advice was to figure out where I wanted to be in the next five years and ten years of my career and accept only those responsibilities that were related in some way to reaching those goals. This meant that instead of accepting random research projects to please senior faculty, I said yes carefully to those projects that led toward my goals. Of course, this meant learning to say no, which is another important life de-stressor.

Dr. Magee gave me great advice, and I have used this principle often to guide my decision-making.

▸ EAVESDROP: *Become a List-Maker*

The word "list" historically comes from the word for listen. List-making is a way to eavesdrop on yourself. On a superficial level, lists help unload our brains. Our short-term memories can hold about seven items at a time, and it takes a lot of mental energy to keep track of everything we need to do. When we write down all the things we have to accomplish, we free up brain power and organize our thoughts instead of letting them swim around chaotically in our heads.

I suggest making several lists. Keep a list of things you must accomplish immediately or within the next couple of days, a list of things to take care of in the next few weeks, and a categorical list of items to address over the long term.

Making lists not only de-clutters your brain and frees up mental energy, but it maximizes your use of "found time." Found time are those 15 minutes you have because your meeting finished early, an appointment cancelled, or you are waiting for your kids to get out of soccer practice. Instead of wondering what you should do next, the list allows you to maximize this time by knowing which phone calls to make, which errand you can squeeze in, or what information you needed to look up off the Internet. Keep your list with you. I keep my "today" list in a little notebook in my pocket so I can pull it out at anytime. You get a lot done without actually adding any more appointments to your day, and you can de-stress at the same time.

List-making gives us back our sense of control. I love crossing items off a list. Yes, I am one of those people who writes chores on a list and crosses them off even when they were not on the list in the first place. It makes me feel like I have accomplished something and gives me added satisfaction. I also don't have to wonder if I have completed a task. If it is crossed off, it is out of my mind.

Get a little help from your friends and family. Laying out the things you need to do in the short term and long term organizes your life in a way that allows you to ask for help. I have come to realize that despite the fact that I like to stay in control and do things myself, in order to stay sane and ultimately reach my goal of a balanced life, I need to ask for help. Instead of keeping everything in my head, making a list lets me delegate. How many times have people asked if they could help you at work or at home and you don't know where to tell them to start? You know you could use a hand but have not organized your thoughts enough to let them help you.

Lists are not all work. Even if you are checking off accomplished tasks right and left, if your lists contain only chores, it can become drudgery. Don't forget to put something fun on your list to look forward to. It can be as simple as a quick call to a friend, meeting your husband for a drink alone, or taking 10 minutes to preview your next vacation destination on the Internet. If you are as thorough as my mother, your daily list will end with, "Go to bed." She has accomplished her day, and her reward is rest.

Finally, lists are not only about the present and future. They are a useful tool for remembering the joy in life, the things that make us happy, accomplishments you are proud of, your good-work list, and your reasons to celebrate. This kind of list can help you pause in a busy life to activate your Bliss.

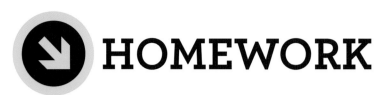

HOMEWORK

Let's take some steps to de-stress your Brain and free yourself to feel Bliss. Exercising your brain via making lists and analyzing them challenges your Brain in a new way and increases the positive effects of exercise on the Brain. Make the following lists:

1. Give Yourself a Break List: What are you going to skip, eliminate, or give yourself permission to let go of?

2. Change Your Loyalties List: What are the top ten products/services/places you consume? Think of ways to minimize the stress of procuring these items by getting them online, delivered, or delegating them to someone else.

3. Stop Creating More Stress List: Think of the ways you personally add to the stress in your life, and then stop it.

4. Do Today List: Prioritize and delegate as possible. Maximize your "found time."

5. Do This Month List: Prioritize. Are there items on this list that are more than three months old? Are they still important?

6. What Makes Me Happy List

7. What Am I Thankful for List

8. Remarkable Times in My Life List

9. Good Work List

10. Relationships I Cherish List

We are social creatures, and with social media and hyper-connectivity we are able to "friend" thousands of people at one time. But how deeply connected can we really be in 140 characters and with 1,000 people? Instead of spending hours reaching out to a multitude of people, make a list of people you will go deep with. Tell them why they are important to you, and foster those relationships verbally and in person.

NOTES

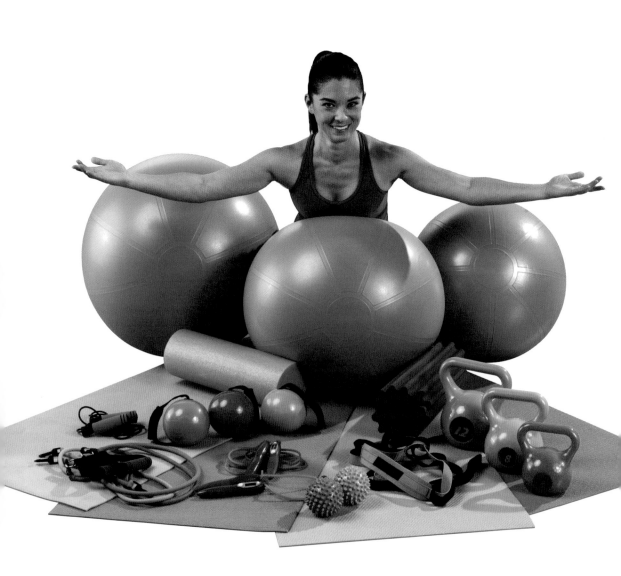

CHAPTER 8

Your Just Rewards

*"Great things are not done by impulse,
but by a series of small things brought together."*
—Vincent Van Gogh

Congratulations, my friend! You have been THRIVE-ing for two months now. Do you realize all that you have accomplished?

You performed the very hard work of getting to know yourself and setting long and short-term goals. You learned, with your Brain and Body, more than 25 total body THRIVE exercises and how to use them in a circuit. Your Brain was de-cluttered by the implementation of list-making, and I hope, by accounting for your past successes and going deep with people you love, you are feeling more Bliss.

Make a concrete list of what you Achieved in the last two months by category. This is, in itself a way to reward your hard work.

How did you do with your first round of goal-setting? Were the goals realistic, attainable? How can you make them more concrete in the next round?

▶ BODY:

1. MOVE: Know Your Numbers

    a. Weight two months ago _____ now_____

    b. Waist two months ago _____ now _____

    c. Hips two months ago _____ now _____

    d. Waist/hip ratio two months ago _____ now _____

    e. Do your clothes fit differently?_____

    f. Are you able to complete the TBT circuits without stopping?

    g. How many days per week are you investing time in MOVE-ing?___

    h. Do you feel more fit?_____

    i. List your favorite exercises:

_____

_____

    j. List your least favorite exercises:

_____

_____

2. EAT:

    a. Which of your eating habits surprised you? _____

    b. Did you adopt the 500 rule? _____

    c. What small substitutions made the most significant changes in your eating habits?_____

_____

_____

▶ BRAINS:

1. THINK:

    a. Did you learn about the stressors in your life?_____

    b. What were several major things you gave yourself a break about?

    _____

    _____

    c. Did you maximize your "found time?"_____

2. FEEL:

    a. Which relationship did you connect/go deep with?

    _____

    b. Did it make you happy to do so?

    _____

    c. How does THRIVE-ing feel now?

    _____

    _____

    _____

    _____

    _____

Log your fitness and nutrition progress into your THRIVE F.A.N. Club page.

What were the major hurdles to your success?

How will you deal with these?

What contributed most greatly to your Achievement?

What do you need to do to go forward in the next two months?

Remember when you were preparing to THRIVE you discussed creating a Vision with several people? Seek them out and tell them how it is going. Give them an update.

Go get your two-month reward. You deserve it! This is your year to THRIVE.

SECTION

③

THRIVE:
Months 3 and 4

"I have learned this, at least, by my experiments; that if one advances confidently in the directions of his dreams, and endeavors to live the life he has imagined, he will meet with a success unexpected in common hours."

—Henry David Thoreau

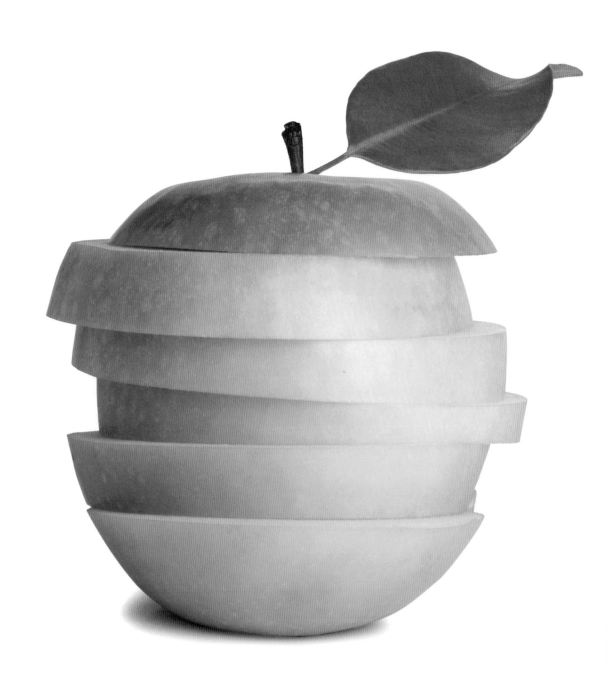

CHAPTER 9

A Vision of Your Bright Future

Whew! Two months down and four to go in your THRIVE-ing journey. Think of what you just accomplished and where we are going next. I hope you feel a renewed confidence in your ability to make small changes that mean a lot to your life.

In the next two months we solidify what you have already learned and crank it up a notch. I am still teaching you very specific methods for THRIVE-ing through MOVE-ing, EAT-ing, THINK-ing, and FEEL-ing, but I'm throwing new challenges at you more often. Why? At this point I know you are committed. I know you can handle more, and I want to prepare you for independence during the fifth and sixth months of our journey.

In the next two months I teach you to keep MOVE-ing to F.A.C.E. your future. We do this by introducing you to the four components of fitness every adult needs to maximize performance and minimize injury—F (flexibility), A (aerobic exercise), C (carrying a load), and E (equilibrium/balance). We use a new set of circuits to challenge your body and make the most of your time investment.

In this section you will also take the time to get to know your food. It is impossible to make the best decisions about what to put in your body without knowing your food. As I was reviewing what I knew about nutrition to write chapter 10, it renewed my commitment to making smart and easy choices in the grocery store. And the next day, I did.

Chapter 11 will continue our discovery of the science behind building brains with exercise and the physical connection between the body and happiness. I suggest tips for staying sharp as you age and more tips for recharging your soul.

These are exciting times ahead. These are also the times, I have found with my patients, when the "new" wears off and we are tempted to do what comes easy instead of what keeps us THRIVE-ing. If you need to take a day off, then take a day off but come right back. You are doing too much good to stop now.

▶ A NEW VISION

Now it is time to set some new goals for this section. Start by briefly writing down your two-month goals from the last section. If you reached your two-month goals, we are ready to take the next steps forward. If you still have things to accomplish from your first set, do not worry—bring the straggling goals along, and we will check them off now.

Proceed now to write your follow-up goals for Months 3 and 4 in each of our four Action/Attitude categories. Both sets should lead you to the goals you set for our six months together. Remember we are breaking down the six-month goals into manageable, smaller components.

MOVE-ing

Two-month goals:

Four-month goals:

Six-month goals:

EAT-ing

Two-month goals:

Four-month goals:

Six-month goals:

▶ ATTITUDE FOCUS FOR YOUR BRAIN AND BLISS

THINK-ing

Two-month goals:

Four-month goals:

Six-month goals:

FEEL-ing

Two-month goals:

Four-month goals:

Six-month goals:

▶ MY GOALS FOR MONTHS 3–4:

✓ **MOVE:** THRIVE-ers will engage their bodies and engage their brains by learning to F.A.C.E. their future with four complete TBT circuits and the tools that prepare them to create their own future workouts.

✓ **EAT:** THRIVE-ers will know their food by understanding the roles of macro-nutrients and micro-nutrients in their daily diets. They will use this knowledge to make simple changes to improve their nutrition.

✓ **THINK:** THRIVE-ers will continue to stimulate brain development via exercise and learn new methods for keeping their brains sharp as they age.

✓ **FEEL:** THRIVE-ers will learn to create happiness in their own space and time.

When I picture THRIVE-ing, I think about taking steps to fortify my body and brain, pushing my personal envelope to Achieve while Renewing my body and mind in the journey. I ask myself the question, "How F.A.R. can I go?" Now I ask you, "How F.A.R. can you go?"

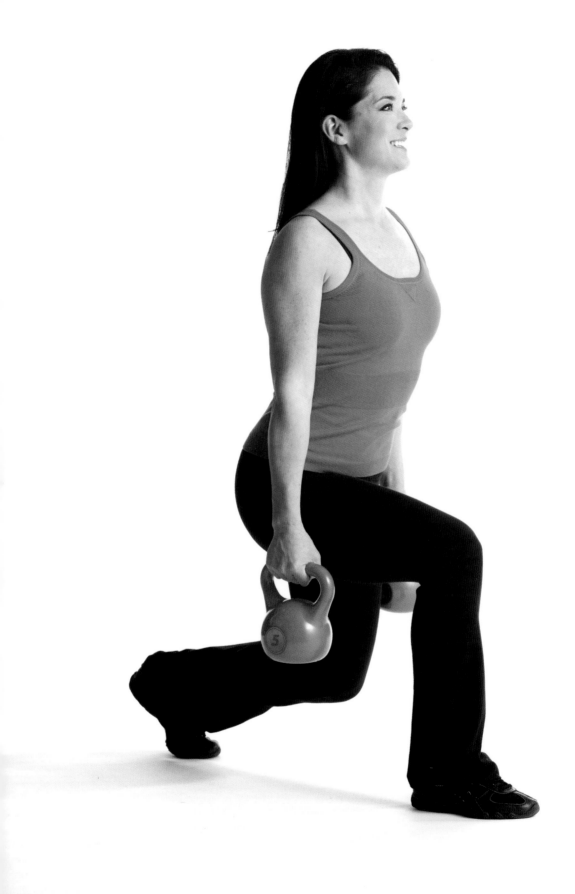

CHAPTER 10

How F.A.R. Can You Go?

"The credit belongs to the man who is actually in the arena; whose face is marred by sweat and blood; who strives valiantly; who errs and comes short again and again because there is no effort without error and shortcoming; who knows the great enthusiasms, the great devotion, spends himself in a worthy cause; who at best knows in the end the triumph of high achievement; and who at worst, if he fails, at least fails while daring greatly, so that his place shall never be with those cold and timid souls who have never tasted victory or defeat."

—Theodore Roosevelt

▶ KEEP MOVE-ING TO F.A.C.E. YOUR FUTURE

We are designed to MOVE! In our body's architecture, we see form following function in every detail, from our two strong legs, meant to propel us forward over a variety of terrains, to our buttocks, intended to slow down momentum and keep us upright.

▶ **STEPS TO MOVE** *Months 3–4*

Step 1: Review the Thrive Skill Summary table. It summarizes all of the exercises you learned in Months 1–2 and will learn in Months 3–4.

Step 2: Review the daily sample schedule for your daily workout. To find out what categories of exercised to do each day follow down the column present for each day of the week. For instance, on Tuesday of Weeks 9–10, you foamroll, DW, do aerobic exercise, and finally equilibrium exercises. To find the exercises in each category for the day, refer to the exercise lists on pp. 130–31. The individual exercises are described on p. 134.

Step 3: Learn the exercise skills listed in each circuit. Use this in your daily workouts.

In chapter 6, you made your first MOVE by learning a dynamic warm-up and two Total Body THRIVE (TBT) circuits. Over the last two months, I hope taking time to THRIVE a little each day has become a habit for you.

Now it is time to keep MOVE-ing and F.A.C.E. your future. I always say that when we become adults in our thirties, forties, fifties, sixties, and beyond, our bodies are unique. They are not merely afterthoughts of what we were before, and we can't just run out the door and exercise recklessly like kids. Our Powerplay needs to be smart, intense, and fun.

Powerplay for adults means staying at the top of your game by focusing on the four components of fitness every adult body needs—F (flexibility), A (aerobic conditioning), C (carrying a load), and E (equilibrium/balance). I introduced you to this philosophy in my first book, *Fitness After 40: How to Stay Strong at Any Age.* Your exercise will now focus on incorporating these total body components. I suggest reading over this entire chapter first to get an overview of our plans and then return here to begin.

▶ HOW TO F.A.C.E. YOUR FUTURE

In Months 3 and 4, I will teach you five additional dynamic warm-up skills and circuits for flexibility, aerobic training, carrying a load, and equilibrium/balance. Learning new skills challenges your body to continue adapting and get stronger. These months build upon the skills and habits you learned in Months 1–2. Our plan is summarized in the Months 3–4 column below.

Total Body THRIVE Skill Summary					
Chapter 6: Make the first MOVE				**Chapter 10: Keep MOVE-ing**	
	Week 1–2	Week 3–4	Week 5–8	Months 3–4	Summary
Dynamic Warm-up	Hip rotations Activator High knee-to-chest lunge	Jumping jacks Sky reach Leg swings-side Leg swings (front/back) Backward lunge/twist			8 TBT skills; Jog 30 yards between each skill
F.A.C.E. your Future					
F (Flexibility)	Foam Rolling			Chest/shoulders Triceps Trunk Trunk twists Hip flexors Piriformis Adductors/ hamstrings Quad Calves	TBT FC (flexibility circuit); stretch AFTER warming up
A (Aerobic exercise)	Walk/run method			Jump rope Walk/run Mini-circuits: kettle swing/ kettle chop/ squat jump (205) Spinning	Use a variety of aerobic exercises to keep your heart rate up

	Week 1–2	Week 3–4	Week 5–8	Months 3–4	Summary
C (Carry a load)					
CC: Core	Plank	Side plank	Mountain climber; Kettle chop	Fire hydrant Plank on ball Side plank with leg raise/swing McGill curl Russian Twist Hip cross overs	10 TBT CC (core circuit)
LE: Butt/hips/legs	Monster walk Prisoner squat	Hip raises Split squat	Half squat with kettle bell; Kettle bell swing; Balance reach; Air plane	Step ups Ball squat Split reverse squat Three-directional lunge Split jump lunge	13 TBT LE (lower extremity) circuit
UE: Upper body/ back	Scaption/ shrug Push-up	RC in four directions W.I.T.Y.	Curl to lunge to press; Back row; Chair dip	Superman Biceps	17 TBT UB (upper body) circuit
E: Equilibrium/ balance					Stork Weighted stork Single leg balance squat (52) Balance reach

By now you know when and how to make time to MOVE. Again, your goal is 2–3 days of TBT skills and 3–5 days per week of aerobic exercise. Each workout is preceded by a dynamic warm-up to get your blood pumping, warm up your muscles, and put you in the best frame of mind. Now we add in F (flexibility circuit) and E (equilibrium training).

The following is a sample schedule for the next two months. Every two weeks I increase the number of days and exercises we use to challenge your body. Initially we begin by adding the flexibility circuit (FC) one day a week and learn new circuits for the core, upper body, and lower body. While you are learning the new exercises, perform sets as described.

In weeks 11–12, we begin combining them in complete circuits. At this point, you perform each exercise for 45 seconds followed by 15 seconds of rest before moving to the next. Gradually we begin to stack these total body THRIVE circuits with the aerobic exercise. Remember, this is a sample schedule. You must make the timing work for you. If you need to skip a day, don't feel bad—just pick up where you left off and keep MOVE-ing.

▶ SAMPLE SCHEDULE

		Mon	Tues	Wed	Thurs	Fri	Sat	Sun	Comments
Week 9–10						Rest		Rest	Five days of exercise, two days of rest; build on chapter 6 exercises with new focused TBT circuits for CC/LE/UB, Flexibility, and Equilibrium
F (Flexibility)									
	Flexibility circuit						x		Following workout
	Foam rolling		x		x		x		Prior to DW/A
A (Aerobic Exercise)									
	DW	x	x	x	x		x		Perform five new DW exercises in this chapter prior to exercise
	Aerobic		x		x		x		Three days
C (Carry a Load)									Three days: perform only the new exercises in this chapter
	TBT	CC		LE	UB				
E (Equilibrium)		x	x	x	x	x	x		Use in life daily

		Mon	Tues	Wed	Thurs	Fri	Sat	Sun	Comments
Week 11–12						Rest		Rest	Wed./Sat. big days; Five days of exercise, two days of rest; Combine exercises in chapter 6 and 10 to form TBT circuits for CC, LE, and UE
F (Flexibility)									
	Flexibility circuit	x		x			x		Following workout
	Foam rolling		x		x		x		Prior to workout
A (Aerobic Exercise)									
	DW	x	x	x	x		x		Combine new DW with the DW exercises learned during Months 1–2 for a total of eight exercises
	Aerobic		x	x	x		x		Four days
C (Carry a Load)									Four days: perform entire circuit of exercises from chapter 6 and chapter 10
	TBT	LE		CC	UE		CC /UE		Four days: perform 1-2 circuits of 45 seconds of exercise with 15 seconds of rest
E (Equilibrium)		x	x	x	x	x	x		
Week 13–14						Rest		Rest	Five days of exercise, 2 days of rest; Stack Aerobic/TBT days
F (Flexibility)									
	Flexibility circuit	x	x	x	x		x		Perform daily following workout
	Foam rolling	x	x	x	x		x		Use as a warm-up prior to DW for problem areas
A (Aerobic Exercise)									
	DW	x	x	x	x		x		Complete eight-exercise circuit but add 30 yards of walking/jogging between each exercise prior to workout
	Aerobic		x	x	x		x		Four days
C (Carry a Load)									
	TBT	UE/ LE		CC	UE/ LE		CC		Four days

		Mon	Tues	Wed	Thurs	Fri	Sat	Sun	Comments
Week 15–16						Rest		Rest	
F (Flexibility)									
	Flexibility circuit	x	x	x	x		x		Daily following exercise
	Foam rolling	x	x	x	x		x		Use as a warm-up prior to DW for problem areas
A (Aerobic Exercise)									
	DW	x	x	x	x		x		Daily prior to exercise. Use eight-exercise circuits with 30 yards of walking/jogging between exercises.
	Aerobic		x		x		x		Intensify aerobic
C (Carry a Load)									
	TBT	UE/ LE/ CC		UE/ LE/ CC			UE/ LE/ CC		TBT stack: choose 10 exercises from each of the three circuits and perform for 45 seconds with 15 seconds of rest in between
E (Equilibrium)		x	x	x	x	x	x		

To challenge yourself to the next level, follow my Go F.A.R. Tips. F.A.R. stands for Fortify, Achieve, Revive, the three pillars of my exercise philosophy.

▶ DYNAMIC WARM-UP II

Just as you did in the first two months, the dynamic warm-up exercises are performed prior to your aerobic and TBT circuit training. The purpose is to get your blood pumping, move your joints through a full range of motion, and activate your muscles.

In Weeks 9–10, learn and warm up with the new exercises detailed in the following pages. Once these are established in your mind and muscles, combine them in an eight-exercise DW circuit.

Finally, in Weeks 11–16, perform the entire DW warm-up circuit but increase the efficacy of the warm-up by walking or jogging 30 yards between each exercise.

▶ DW EXERCISES

Jumping Jacks: Cardio Warm-Up

1. Engage your core and roll your shoulders back by squeezing your shoulder blades together.

2. Explode to a jumping jack position and immediately return to the starting position.

3. Do 20 reps.

 Go F.A.R. Tip: **Hold a THRIVE toning ball in each hand.**

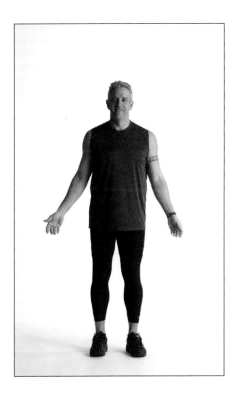 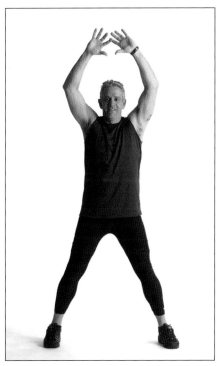

Sky Reach: Upper Back Mobility

1. Engage your core and bend forward from the hips until your chest is parallel to the floor with your knees slightly bent and your feet shoulder-width apart.

2. Begin with your arms hanging straight down in front of your shoulders.

3. Rotate your chest to the right from your waist and reach with your right hand as high as you can.

4. Return to the starting position and repeat to the left. This is one rep.

5. Do 20 reps.

 Reach for your toes between reps.

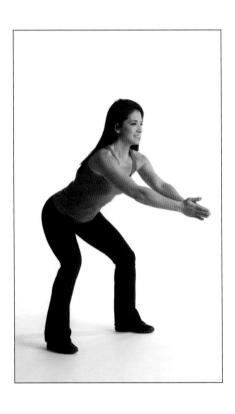 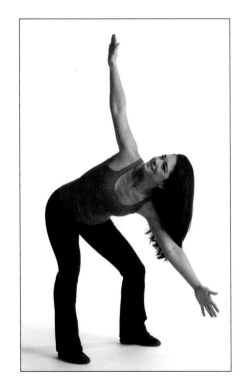

Leg Swings to Side: Hip Mobility, Buttock Activation

1. Engage your core and balance on one leg.

2. Gently swing one leg in front and across your body and then out to the side like a pendulum 10 times.

3. Switch to the opposite side.

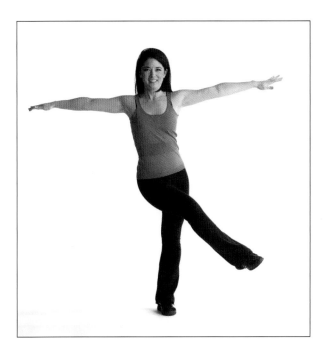

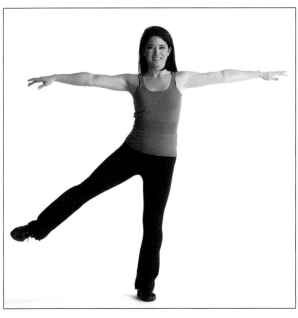

Leg Swings to Front/Back: Hip Mobility, Hip Flexor, Buttock Activation

1. Engage your core and balance on one leg.

2. Gently swing one leg front to back 10 times.

3. Switch to the opposite side.

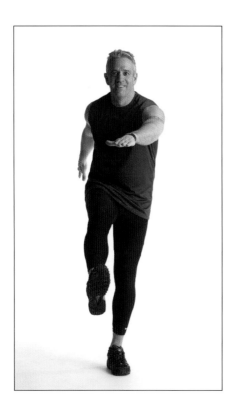
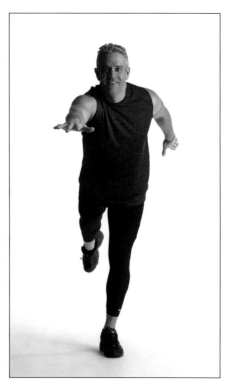

Backward Lunge and Twist: Core, Buttock, Quad Activation, Trunk Rotation

1. Engage your core, and keep your trunk upright.

2. Step back with your right leg and lower your body into a lunge.

3. While stepping back, rotate your arms to the right.

4. Keep your trunk upright and your front knee over your ankle.

5. Alternate legs stepping backward.

6. Do 20 reps.

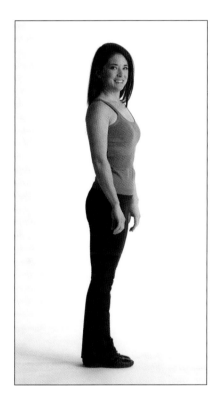 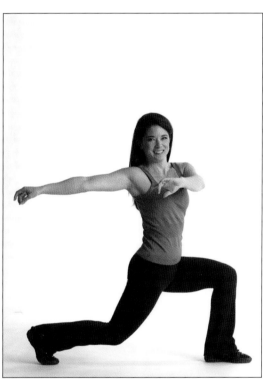

▶ **F** = *Flexibility Facts*

As we age, our muscles and tendons naturally become shorter. This leads to abnormal muscle firing, decreased joint range of motion, and an increased potential for injury. We can prevent these changes by stretching daily. Yes, I said daily. It does not take long, and you may perform stretches anywhere, not just in the gym.

The following series of pictures demonstrates the total body F (Flexibility) circuit. Some of the exercises use a flexibility strap to aid in the stretch, while others use only your body. As with the other total body exercises you have learned, always engage your core prior to beginning.

Perform this static flexibility circuit *after* the A (Aerobic) and/or C (Carry a Load) TBT circuit training when your body is warmed up and your muscles are supple. The stretches should feel like a gentle pull, not sharp pain. Hold all stretches for 30 seconds. Toward the end of the 30 seconds, you will feel your muscles relax more and give you more of a stretch. Remember, no bouncing or ballistic stretching.

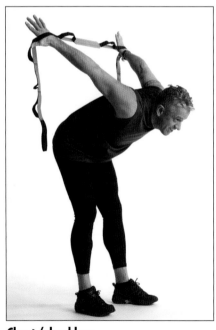

Chest/shoulders

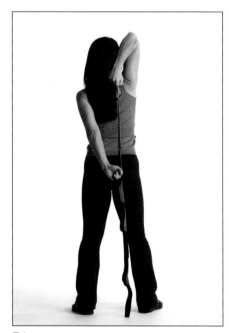

Triceps

Demonstrated with the THRIVE flexibility strap available exclusively at Dick's Sporting Goods stores.

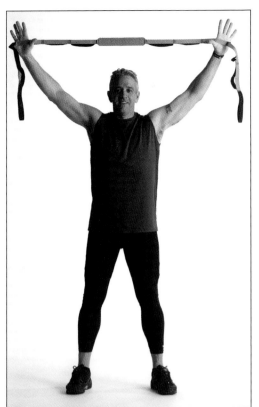
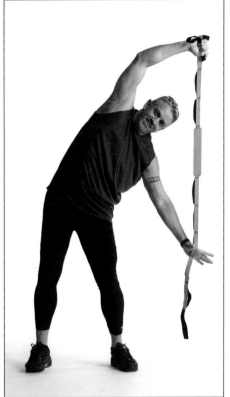

Trunk

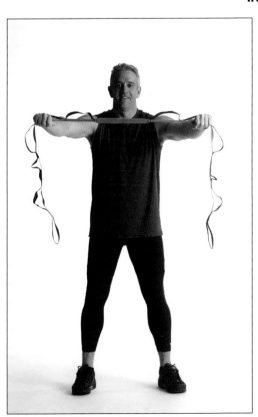
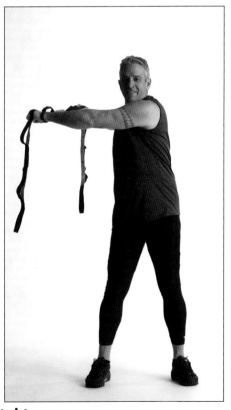

Trunk twists

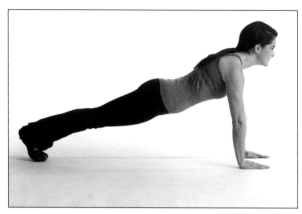

Hip flexors

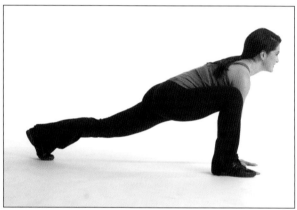

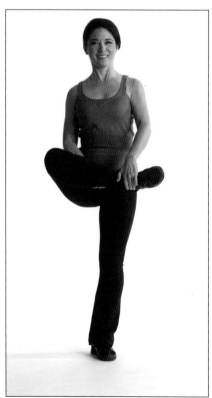

Piriformis

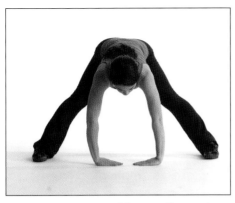

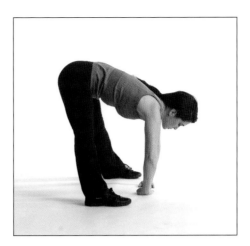

Adductors/hamstrings

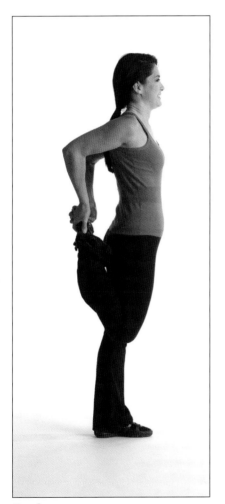

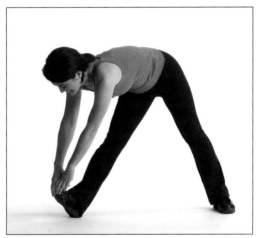

Calves

Quad

▶ **A** = *Aerobic Exercise*

In our very busy lives, how do we get the most out of our workouts in the least amount of time? Many new studies show that aerobic interval training—where aerobic exercise is performed at high intensity (90 percent MHR) for short bursts of time followed by short rest periods—is much more effective than continuous moderate exercise (70 percent MHR) for preventing and treating metabolic syndrome (high blood pressure, diabetes, high cholesterol, and central obesity) and cardiovascular disease, and it can improve aerobic fitness.

A study published in *Circulation* found that aerobic intensity training (AIT)—with a 10-minute warm-up followed by four four-minute intervals of intense walking/running at 90 percent of MHR, and each followed by a three-minute active recovery at 70 percent MHR, for a total of 40 minutes of exercise—was more effective at increasing aerobic capacity and delivery of oxygen to the body than longer periods of moderate exercise. AIT also improved the amount of blood the heart pumped with each beat (stroke volume) and muscle efficiency. The study found that while both groups lost weight, the AIT group was more protected from cardiovascular disease and death. This indicates that although targeting both the risk factors of weight loss and increased aerobic capacity is optimal, if you have to prioritize, choose to become fit before thin.

A subsequent study comparing AIT with three-times-per-week strength training (ST) and a combination of both found that ST and ST with AIT had significant positive effects on improving aerobic capacity and decreasing the risks of chronic disease.

The A (aerobic) exercise prescribed in Chapter 6 was designed to get you MOVE-ing. At this point you should know what works for you and what doesn't. In the next two months, we will fine-tune your aerobic exercise to maximize your performance and minimize injury.

One way we do this is to increase the time and intensity of your aerobic experience. Remember, although both are important for overall health, my priority for you as a physician is to be fit. Thin will follow.

In Weeks 9–10, warm up with 10 minutes of our dynamic warm-up exercises. Next, perform 25–30 minutes of AIT followed by 10 minutes of cool down, including flexibility, for a total of 45–50 minutes of exertion. The AIT pattern should include three to four minutes of aerobic exercise at 90 percent MHR followed by one to two minutes of recovery at 70 percent MHR.

If you are new to exercise, begin these intervals on a treadmill or elliptical machine equipped with a heart-rate monitor to teach your body what this level of exertion feels like. Although many people find running on a treadmill monotonous, this type of speed-play can actually be fun as you seemingly compete against yourself during the intense phase and get to reward yourself with a short recovery each cycle.

After 10 weeks of interval-type aerobic exercise (we began this approach in Months 1–2), you will feel in tune with how your body responds to increased aerobic demand and the AIT seems easier than when you started. The beauty of AIT is that at any moment you can ramp it up by increasing the AIT time and decreasing the recovery time.

Another way to maximize your performance and minimize injury (and to prevent boredom) is to try new ways to play. Your Body doesn't care how you get your heart rate up, just that you do. In Weeks 11–12, continue to do AIT using a walk/run method one to two days per week, but throw in some aerobic variety on the other A (aerobic) days. Use the same time/ intensity pattern, but perform the aerobic exercise via different method, such as jumping rope, spinning, rowing, stair climbing, swimming, jumping jacks, etc. Really, anything will work.

By the end of 12 weeks, you will definitely be noticing changes in your Body. What I'm teaching you will seem easier, your clothes will fit differently, and you will have more stamina for daily activity. You may notice, however, that while you were caring for your Body, your Brain is thinking more clearly, you are solving problems more easily (probably during your aerobic workouts), and you will feel the Bliss of accomplishment. You are doing great.

Finally, in Weeks 13–16, try getting really creative with your cardio work. Continue with the methods that have worked for you in the prior three months, but really mix it up now by doing aerobic mini-circuits. Simply choose three to four TBT circuit exercises and string them together into mini circuits. Perform each exercise rapidly, but with good form, for one to two minutes and then rest for 15 seconds. Make sure to monitor your heart rate to ensure you are maximizing your effort.

Sample Mini-Circuits

✓ **Kettle bell swing, kettle bell chop, squat jump**
✓ **Split jump, vertical jump, alternating forward lunge**

▶ C = *Carry a Load*

In my F.A.C.E. approach to total body fitness, C stands for Carry a Load. By this I mean resistance training. I specifically do not call this weight lifting, and you will never see a weight machine in my TBT circuits. In life, your body never sits statically and pushes weight in one direction without gravity. Why would you spend time and energy training your body to do something it never does in reality? There is nothing more frustrating than spending countless hours working out only to realize you haven't made any progress.

My TBT circuits work your body in the same way you use your body every day. We harness the pull of gravity, the ground reactive forces, to push back every time you land and build power through three planes of motion.

The new circuits build on the exercises you learned in chapter 6. Look back up at the table on page 123. You can perform the new exercises in the order they appear going down the Week 3–4 summary column or by following the exercises across the row for each specific circuit focus, core circuit (CC), upper extremity (UE), and lower extremity (LE).

This may seem like a lot of variation, but the fact is your body hates predictability and will respond to change by becoming more efficient and strong.

During Weeks 9–10, you will learn and perform only the new exercises in the TBT circuits for core (CC), upper body (UE), and lower body (LE). Do each set once per week, as suggested in the sample schedule, while your brain and body learn them. Perform two sets of the exercises during these weeks. Remember that until your muscle memory for each new exercise kicks in, you may feel awkward. Don't be discouraged—every time you perform the moves, they get easier.

In Weeks 11–12, I will teach you circuit training. This may be a completely new way to train for you, but it increases the intensity of your work and challenges your muscles by adding the exercises you learned in chapter 6 to your new regimen. You will do each body area (CC, LE, UE) once per week, and on Saturday you will step it up by stacking two circuits. Instead of doing sets of the exercises, as in the previous two weeks, you now complete them in a circuit by doing each for 45 intense seconds followed by 15 seconds of rest. The goal is to keep your heart rate up and keep you moving the entire time. You are going to have so much fun. Now this is Powerplay.

Finally in Weeks 13–16, we simply continue performing the TBT circuits you now perform easily and increase the intensity by an extra day of C (carrying a load) per week and stacking the CC, LE, and UE TBT circuits on the same day. Perform each of the 10 exercises from the CC, LE, and UE circuits for 45 seconds followed by 15 seconds of rest. This adds up to about 30 minutes of intense and fun work.

▶ C: CORE CIRCUIT (CC)

Fire Hydrant: Core Stability

1. Begin on your hands and knees with your hips directly over your knees and your shoulders directly over your hands. Engage your core, and keep your back straight.

2. Your knees and hands should be shoulder-width apart.

3. Keeping your back straight, raise your right leg as close as you can to your chest.

4. Raise your right leg to the side with your knee bent.

5. Straighten your leg back until it is in line with your trunk.

6. This is one rep. Perform 10 reps on each leg.

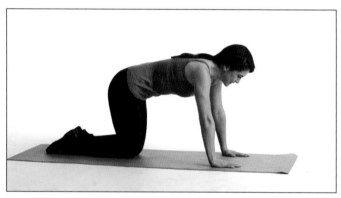

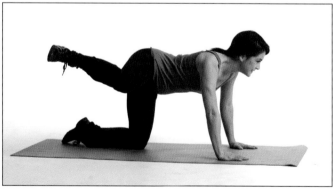

Plank on Ball: Core Stability, Upper Body Strength

1. Place your feet and shins on an exercise ball.

2. Get into a push-up position but bend your elbows and place weight on your forearms instead of your hands.

3. Lower your buttocks until your back is flat and your body is in a straight line from ankles to shoulders. Engage your core by pulling your navel toward your spine and pushing down like you were going to be punched in the gut. Make sure your butt is not sticking up or sinking down.

4. Hold for 30 seconds and work up to two minutes. Remember to breathe.

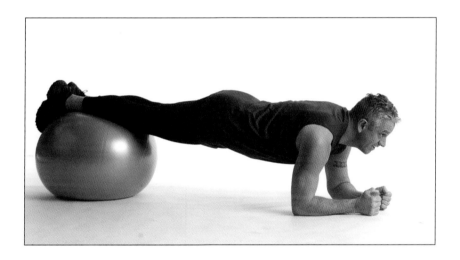

Side Plank with Leg Raise/Swing: Core Stability, Pliometrics

1. Lie on your side and rise up onto your elbow. Place your weight on your forearms and the side of your lower foot. Engage your core and squeeze your butt.

2. Raise your trunk off the floor and lower your buttocks until your body is in a straight line from ankles to shoulders. Make sure your butt is not sticking up or sinking down. Your shoulder should be directly over your elbow.

3. Raise your top leg up as high as you can

4. Hold for 30 seconds and work up to two minutes. Remember to breathe.

 When you can hold the side plank for 60 seconds, challenge your core more by forcing it to maintain stability with motion. Raise the top leg up slightly and move it forward and back while maintaining your plank position.

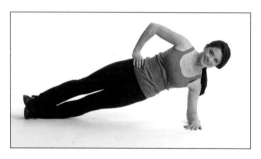 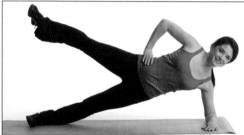

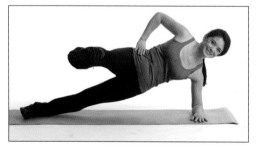 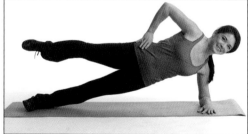

McGill Curl: Core stability, Lower Back Pain Prevention

1. Lay flat on the floor with your left knee bent and right knee straight.

2. Support your lower back with your palms under the small of your back.

3. Keep you chin pointing forward and raise your head and shoulders off the floor without flexing your lower spine.

4. Remember to exhale when you raise your shoulders and inhale as your lower them.

5. Do 20–30 reps.

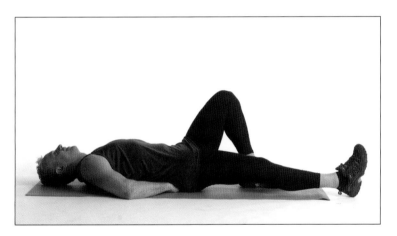

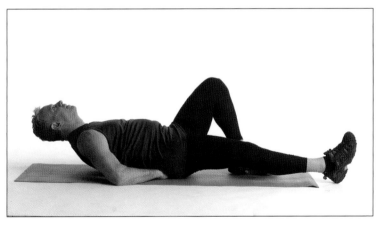

Russian Twist: Oblique Core Stabilization, Hips, Lower Back Pain Prevention

1. Engage your core and sit with your trunk 45 degrees off the floor. Keep your knees bent and feet flat.

2. Extend your arms, palms together, in front of your body.

3. Rotate to the right with your arms and trunk as far as you can.

4. Switch and rotate to the left as far as you can. This is one rep.

5. Do 20 reps.

Go F.A.R. Tip: **Increase the difficulty of this move by holding THRIVE toning balls or a THRIVE kettle bell in your arms.**

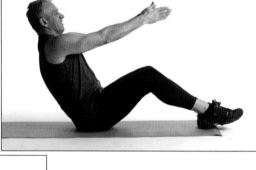

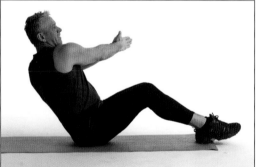

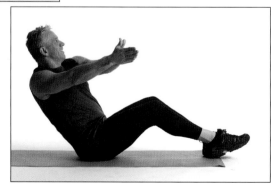

Hip Crossovers: Core Stability, Trunk Rotation

1. While lying on the floor, raise your hips and knees until they are bent 90 degrees. Engage your core and balance by extending your arms out to the sides.

2. Lower your legs to the floor to the right while keeping your shoulders on the floor. You will feel a stretch in your core and lower back but not pain.

3. Cross over your hips to the opposite side. This is one rep.

4. Do 10 reps.

 Go F.A.R. Tip: **Add difficulty by squeezing a THRIVE exercise ball between your thighs and calves.**

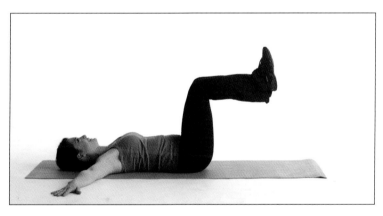

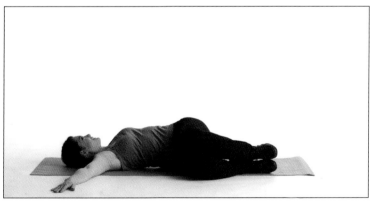

▶ C: LOWER EXTREMITY, BUTT/HIP/ LEG CIRCUIT (LE)

Step-Ups: Butt, Quad, Hamstring

1. Place your left foot firmly on a step or platform that allows your knee to bend 90 degrees or less.

2. Engage your core and push your body up onto the step with your weight on your left heel.

3. Return to the starting position.

4. Perform 10 reps.

5. Switch to the right leg after completing sets with the left.

Go F.A.R. Tip: **Hold a THRIVE toning ball or light kettle bell in each hand.**

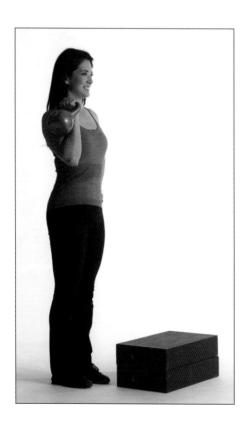
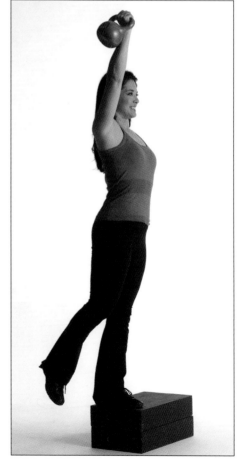

Ball Squat: Butt, Core, Vastus Medialis

1. Place a toning ball or a light medicine ball between your knees.

2. Engage your core and squat down until your knees are bent over your ankles approximately 60 degrees.

3. Squeeze your knees together and hold for three seconds.

4. Return to starting position.

5. Do two sets of 10 reps.

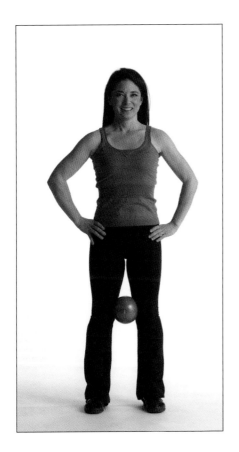
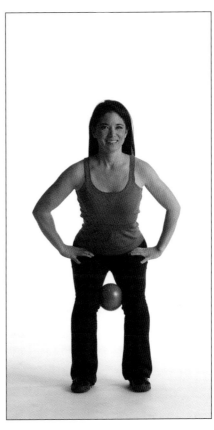

Split Reverse Squat: Butt, Core, Hip Flexor Stretch

1. Engage your core and stand with your feet together.

2. Lunge back with your right foot.

3. Keep the weight on your left heel.

4. Tuck your right buttocks under and feel the engagement of your hip flexor.

5. Hold three seconds and return to starting position.

6. Do two sets of 10 reps.

 Hold kettle bells in your hands and press them above your shoulders as you lunge back.

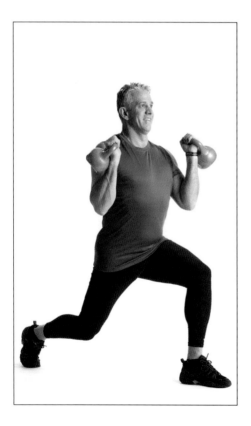 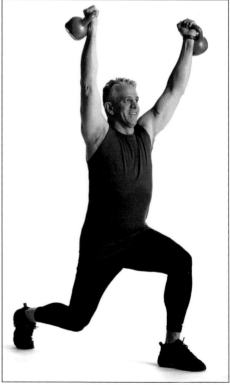

Lunge Matrix in Three Planes of Motion: Core, Butt, Quads, Hamstrings

In this lunge matrix, you will lunge to the front, side and back (12:00, 3:00, and 6:00 on a clock face). Each lunge direction is driven by your arms moving in three planes of motion (front, side, rotation).

1. To start, lunge forward to 12:00 with your left leg and drive your arms straight overhead.

2. Pause and return to the starting position.

3. Lunge to 12:00 again, but drive your arms to the side over your left leg.

4. Finally, repeat the lunge but rotate your arms through your trunk over your left leg.

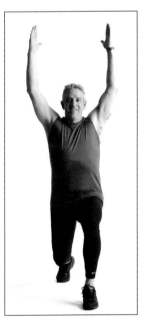
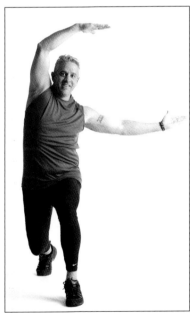
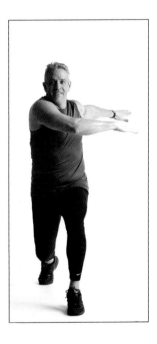

5. Repeat step three but with your lunge to 3:00. Remember to drive the lunges with your arms to the front, side, and in rotation.

6. Repeat step three but with your lunge to 6:00. Again, remember to drive the lunges with your arms to the front, side, and in rotation.

7. When you complete the lunges with the left leg, repeat the series while lunging with the right leg.

The three lunges in three planes of motion on each leg is one matrix or 18 lunges!

Split Jump Lunge: Core, Butt, Plio

1. Keeping your trunk upright, engage your core and lower your body into a split squat with your left leg back.

2. Explode up into the air with both feet off the ground and switch your right leg to back.

3. Land in a split squat with your left leg front.

4. Do 20 reps.

 Hold a THRIVE toning ball or kettle bell in each hand.

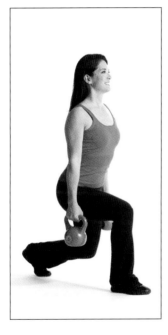 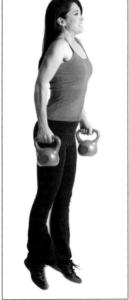 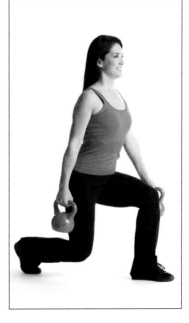

▶ C: UPPER EXTREMITY, UPPER BODY/BACK CIRCUIT (UE)

Supermans: Upper Back, Core

1. While laying on your stomach, brace your core.

2. Extend your arms forward.

3. Raise your arms and legs off the floor simultaneously.

4. Pause and hold for three seconds.

5. Repeat 10 times.

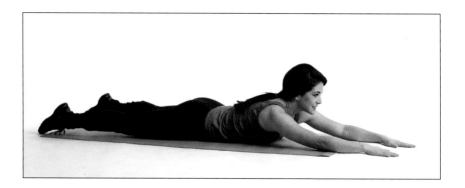

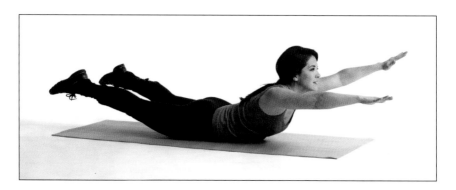

Split Squat with Weight: Upper Body, Quads, Calves, Core, Butt

1. Hold THRIVE toning balls or kettle bells in your hands extended down to your sides.

2. Stand with your left foot in front of your right in a staggered stance with your front knee slightly bent and your weight on the heel of the front foot and toes of the back.

3. Engage your core and squeeze your butt.

4. Slowly lower your body until your hip is parallel to your front knee. Your front knee should be over your ankle and the back knee nearly touching the floor. Keep your torso upright.

5. Pause in this position while squeezing your butt and rotating your hips slightly forward.

6. Press kettle bells, toning balls, or hand weights over head and hold.

7. Push back up to starting position.

8. Do 10 reps on each side.

Biceps: Biceps, Upper Back

1. While holding free weights or THRIVE kettle bells in your hands, stand with your feet shoulder-width apart and brace your core.

2. Keep your palms forward.

3. Keep your elbows next to your body and your upper arms still, then bend your elbows to curl the weight up toward your shoulders.

4. Pause at the top and slowly lower them back to starting position with arms completely straight.

5. Do two sets of 10. Repeat on opposite side.

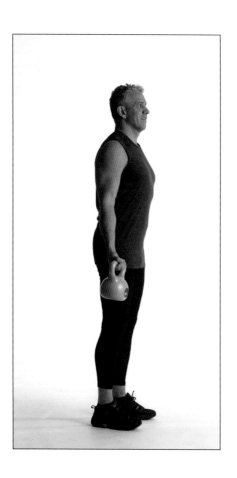 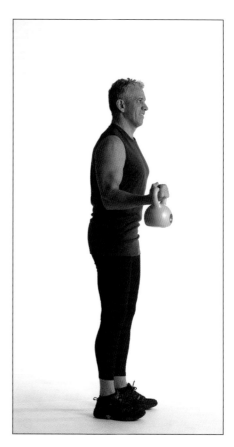

Triceps: Triceps, Upper Back

1. Engage your core and bend forward at the waist, keeping your back straight.

2. Hold a THRIVE toning ball or kettle bell in your right hand.

3. Keeping your elbow close to your side, extend your elbow until straight by flexing your triceps.

4. Hold for three seconds and release.

5. Perform two sets of 10 on each side.

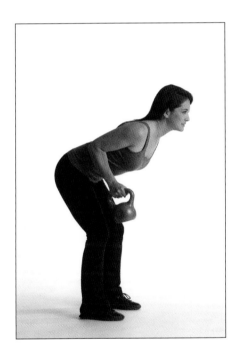
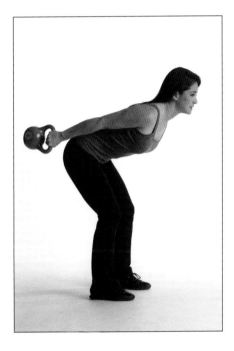

▶ E = *Equilibrium and Balance*

The final component of F.A.C.E.-ing your future is E—equilibrium and balance. After the age of 25 the connections between our brains and muscles begin to become less accurate, leading to declines in proprioception (position sense) and balance as we age. The good news is that these neuromuscular pathways can be retrained with minimal daily attention.

Maintaining our balance is important for maximizing performance and minimizing injury but more important for preventing the falls that can break our wrists and hips and devastate our lives.

▶ HOW DO I KNOW IF MY BALANCE STINKS?

In a safe place, engage your core and stand on one foot. When you are steady, carefully close your eyes. If your balance is adequate you should be able to hold this position for 22 seconds without tipping over. The shorter the amount of time you can balance, the "older" your balance is.

- ✓ **22 seconds = 20 years old**
- ✓ **15 seconds = 30 years old**
- ✓ **7.2 seconds = 40 years old**
- ✓ **3.7 seconds = 50 years old**
- ✓ **Less than 2 seconds = 60 years old**

Fitting equilibrium and balance training into your already busy day is easy. Do not set aside special time to do this—instead, be productive in your down time. (Remember the "found time" I talked about in chapter 7?) Practice these balance moves at various times, such as between sets of your TBT circuits, while brushing your teeth in the morning, while talking on the phone at the office, or even while standing at the bus stop. The equilibrium exercises in this chapter do not require any special equipment and can be performed anytime and anywhere.

Perform several of these balance exercises daily. I fit these exercises into my day by demonstrating them to my patients several times a day or doing the stork while talking on the phone. Nothing so important has ever been this easy.

Stork

1. Engage your core and stand with your feet slightly apart.

2. Raise one leg off the ground while keeping your arms at your sides.

3. Maintain this position for 30 seconds while you go about your normal standing activity (e.g., brushing teeth, talking on the phone, between exercise sets, etc.)

4. Switch legs and hold for 30 additional seconds.

5. Perform several times per day.

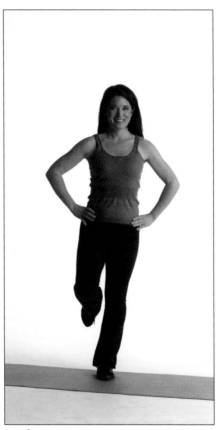

Stork

Weighted Stork

Once the standard stork is easy for you, increase the level of difficulty and therefore your balance skills by holding THRIVE toning balls or kettle bells in your hands. Challenge your balance by doing the stork while swinging your arms like you are running or by standing on a folded bath towel or soft carpet. You can also do the stork or weighted stork standing on a bosu ball.

Balance Reach: Quads, Core, Balance

1. Engage your core and stand with your feet together and hands on your hips.

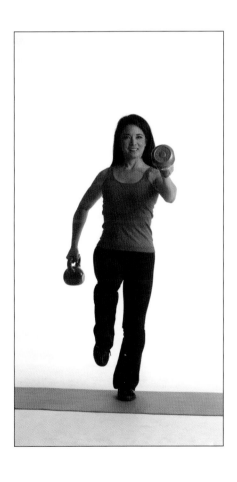
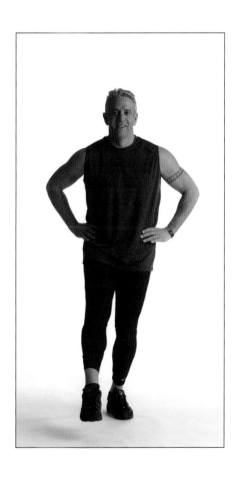

2. Imagine you are standing in the center of a clock. Reach forward with your right toe toward 12:00, and slightly bend your left knee. Keep your hips level and your back straight.

3. Pause and return to a standing position. Repeat to 12:00 10 times.

4. Repeat balance reach to 3:00 to the side and 6:00 to the back with the right leg.

5. Switch sides and repeat balance reach sequence with the left leg.

6. Increase the balance challenge by swinging your arms forward and back or by holding THRIVE toning balls in your arms while you swing.

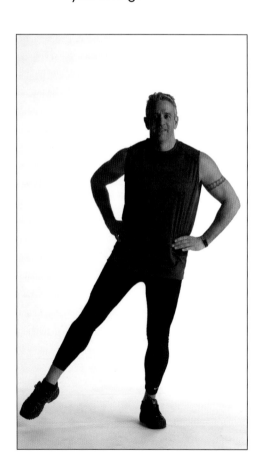 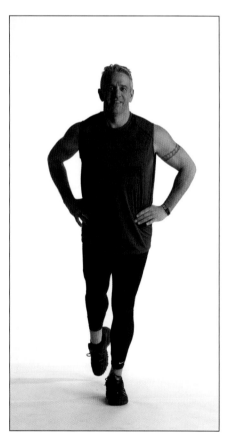

▶ KEEP MOVE-ING AND F.A.C.E. YOUR FUTURE

By the end of this chapter you will know a large menu of exercises for strengthening your entire body and the four important components of fitness for THRIVE-ing adults. The sample schedule may seem overwhelming, but take it day by day. I have spelled out the areas to cover each day. General tips to remember include:

1. Begin each workout day with the THRIVE dynamic warm-up.

2. The foam roller is an excellent way to warm up problem areas before or during the dynamic warm-up.

3. After warming up, perform A (aerobic) or C (carry a load) exercises with the TBT circuits.

4. Perform the static flexibility circuit *after* your workout when your muscles are warm. You may also foam roll problem areas at the end.

5. Fit the Equilibrium exercises into each and every day.

6. If you are short on time, choose five of the circuit exercises from each TBT circuit and perform each for 45 seconds followed by 15 seconds of rest. You can cover a total body workout in about 15 minutes. If you do 5–10 minutes of dynamic warm-up before and five minutes of cool down after, you are out the door in 30 minutes.

▶ EATING TO THRIVE

In chapter 6, we started simply. You learned to know yourself and your eating habits. You learned the 500 Rule and how to make simple changes that mean a lot. Now we take the next step and learn about our food.

Sometimes we have a love/hate relationship with food. Sometimes we love it too much, and sometimes we feel like it is the enemy. The fact is, food is not the enemy but it is powerful, and how we use it can change our health and our lives. The goal in this chapter is to teach you to THRIVE by knowing your food.

▶ KNOWING THE BIG GUNS:
Macro-Nutrients

The Skinny on Carbs

How did carbohydrates get such a bad rap? Sometimes we are led to believe that if you are not a marathon runner, carbs are your enemy. Actually, carbs are the major energy source for your body during activity. Your brain is entirely dependent on carbs for its fuel.

Carbohydrates are simple molecules made of three elements—carbon, hydrogen, and oxygen—linked together by weak bonds. Carbs are made of sugar, the most simple of which, glucose, is the body's primary energy source and is the sugar in the blood. When single sugar molecules are strung together like pearls on a necklace, they form complex carbohydrate types of sugar.

Common Simple-Molecule Sugars
Glucose: blood sugar
Fructose: fruit sugar

Common Double-Molecule Sugars
Sucrose: table sugar
Lactose: milk sugar
Maltose: starch/plant sugar

Our body uses the sugar contained in carbohydrates differently. The simple sugar, glucose, is our primary fuel. It is the sugar that circulates in the blood, and eating glucose raises your blood sugar the fastest. However, another simple sugar, fructose, doesn't spike blood sugar at all but is broken down by the liver into glucose and stored as glycogen for future use. When the sugar storehouse is full, the extra sugar is saved in the form of fat.

Complex carbohydrates contain multiple simple sugar molecules linked together. Starch, the complex sugar found in plants, is readily broken down directly into glucose and is a great energy source. Fiber, the structural sugar that makes up plant stems and leaves, is non-digestible. Although it adds no energy to the fire, it slows absorption of starch and prevents a spike in blood sugar while taking up space in your stomach and leaving you with a full feeling. Fiber is, therefore, great for portion control because you feel full without getting stuffed with absorbable sugar.

The recommended daily dose of carbohydrates is 45–65 percent of total calories consumed, or about 130 grams per day. This number increases if you are training for athletic events and burning more energy. Each gram of carbohydrates contains four calories.

▶ THE GLYCEMIC INDEX:
Crash and Burn

The Glycemic Index is a measure of the effect of carbohydrates on blood glucose levels and insulin production. Easily digestible foods containing high levels of simple sugars cause a rapid spike in circulating blood sugar. This signals the pancreas to release insulin in order to absorb the glucose. This works well unless the pancreas overshoots insulin secretion, which it commonly does, providing too much transportation of the glucose out of the blood. This causes the blood glucose to fall rapidly and leaves you feeling tired, cranky, shaky, and sometimes lightheaded. This precipitous drop spurs a carb crave three to four hours after a high-carb meal and sends you straight the refrigerator for more carbs that are high on the Glycemic Index. Usually, high-index foods also contain a lot of fat and calories, which can set you up for a cycle of overindulging. Filling our meals and snacks with low-index foods and protein will help stop the blood sugar madness. The following table gives examples of foods in the high, moderate, and low-index categories. Notice that some of the high-index foods are obviously high in glucose, such as ice cream. However, some in the high category are more healthy. The caution is to mix up your intake and eat carbs with protein and fat to slow down absorption.

Glycemic Index Foods		
The Good, the Bad, and the Ugly		
LOW	**Moderate**	**High**
Milk	Sponge cake	Cake
Yogurt	Pita	Pastry
Rice bran	Brown/white rice	Candy
Lentils	Barley peas	English muffins
Apricots	Candy bars	Raisins
Multigrain bread	Mango	Chips
Citrus fruits	Kiwi	Sucrose
Apples	Basmati rice	White bread
Tomatoes	Buckwheat	Millet
Pears	Sweet potatoes	Couscous
Plums	PowerBar	Honey/syrup
Beans	Banana	Carrots
Tomato juice	Whole wheat	Pretzels
Chickpeas	Bran cereal	Barley bread
Bran cereal	Citrus juice	Watermelon
Nuts	Oatmeal	Ice cream
Peaches	Grapes	Sports drinks
Hummus	Tortillas	Sports goo
	Pasta	Rye bread
	Corn	Bagels
	Crackers	Cold cereal
		Pancakes
		Potatoes

Adapted from "Sports Nutrition for Coaches," Human Kinetics, Leslie Bonci, MPH, RD

Proteins Are All the Rage

Protein is the building block of the body and vitally important for building and repairing muscle, strengthening the immune system, keeping bones healthy, and making blood. It is also a component in hormone, enzyme, and antibody synthesis, and it raises your metabolism. Although protein can also be used as a source of energy for activity, it is used less than fat or carbs. In addition, protein is digested slowly, leaving you feeling full longer.

Protein is built from individual amino acids, which are molecules composed of the elements carbon, nitrogen, hydrogen, and sulfur. Of the 22 amino acids, our bodies make only 12 of them. The remaining 10 we must eat. The most complete sources of amino acids are meat, dairy foods, and eggs. Many other foods contain amino acids and protein, but only these three contain all the essential amino acids. Everywhere you look there are bottles and bars packed with amino acid supplements and protein. The current data supporting use of amino acid supplement remains inconclusive, so protein from whole foods remains the best source.

Approximately 10 to 35 percent of our daily calories should come from protein, and about one gram contains nine calories. All meat, beef, birds, and fish contain the same amount of protein per ounce. One serving of meat is roughly the size of an iPhone or a deck of cards. Plan on protein as part of every meal.

Fat Is Not an Enemy!

Believe it or not, fat is essential for heart health, blood pressure regulation, hair and skin health, hormone production, and endurance exercise. Several key vitamins—such as A, D, and E—are fat soluble and are absorbed best when consumed with fat. The problem is that in our environment of abundant food, we eat more than our bodies need and we are not smart about which fats we put in our bodies.

Fat is built of fatty acids containing carbon, hydrogen, and oxygen. Fatty acids come in three varieties: saturated, monounsaturated, and polyunsaturated. The more saturated the molecule is with hydrogen molecules, the more solid the fat is at room temperature and the worse it is for your health.

The Good: Monounsaturated and Polyunsaturated Fats

Make the wise choice to eat monounsaturated fats. These plant-based fats decrease the risk of heart disease by reducing bad cholesterol levels, minimizing the feeling of hunger, and supporting memory. Olive oil has become increasingly popular as a source of "good fat" and is mainly composed of Oleic acid, also known as Omega 9. Good sources of monounsaturated fats include nuts, olives, avocados, and sunflower and pumpkin seeds.

Polyunsaturated fats include Omega 6 and Omega 3 fats. Both decrease the risk of heart disease, and Omega 3 is a powerful anti-inflammatory. Omega 3 has received the most attention of late and include EPA, DHA, and ALA. EPA and DHA are found in a variety of foods but mostly in fatty fish. Good sources of Omega 6 polyunsaturated fats include corn oil, safflower oil, sunflower oil, soybean oil, and olive oil. Sources of Omega 3 polyunsaturated fats include fatty fish, flaxseed oil, walnuts, and soybean oil.

The Bad: Saturated and Trans fats

Saturated fats are solid at room temperature and should be avoided in large amounts. Both saturated and trans fats are correlated with increased risk of heart disease. Examples of these bad fats include butter, whole milk, cheese, cream, coconut oil, margarine, and the fat on meat or lard.

The Dietary Guideline for Americans 2005 recommend 20–35 percent of daily calories come from fat. This is further broken down to 10 percent from each type of fat.

The Micro-Nutrients

Called micro because we require only small amounts per day, these vitamins and minerals actually play a big role in many of our body's vital functions. A balanced diet of whole foods will provide us with most of what we need. If you are like so many busy people I care for, myself included, you may not always get enough. That's when a simple multi-vitamin really maximizes your body's storehouse. The table on the next page summarizes the Recommended Dietary Allowances for both the Macro and Micro-Nutrients from the National Institute of Medicine. Use it as a guide for getting what you need.

▶ FILL UP WITHOUT FILLING OUT

1. Eat green and leafy all the time. You won't gain weight, and you will cover your vitamin and mineral needs.

2. Eat protein with every meal. Protein digests slowly and will keep you feeling full longer.

3. Eat healthy fats. Your body needs fat, but you must choose the mono and polyunsaturated versions for the most benefit with the least bad qualities.

4. Cut added sugars, and minimize foods with ingredients you can't pronounce.

5. Nix your membership in the Clean Plate Club. Listen to your body instead. Stop eating when you begin to feel full, not when you have to unbutton your clothes.

6. Don't skip a meal. This makes your body think it is starving so your metabolism slows to conserve energy.

7. Remember what you eat is important. It's a waist line—not a waste line.

Sex		Women			Men			
Age		30-50	50-70	>70	30-50	50-70	>70	Function and Source
Macro-Nutrients	See previous explanations							
	Water (L/day)	2.7	2.7	2.7	3.7	3.7	3.7	
	Carbs (g/day)	130	130	130	130	130	130	
	Fiber (g/day)	25	21	21	38	30	30	
	Linoleic acid (g/day)	12	11	11	17	14	14	
	A-linolenic acid (g/day)	1.1	1.1	1.1	1.6	1.6	1.6	
	Protein (g/day) *	1 g/lbs. of desired body weight per day						
Micro-Nutrients								
	Vitamin A (ug/day)	700	700	700	900	900	900	Immune function; carrots, sweet potatoes
	Vitamin C (mg/day)	70	70	70	90	90	90	Immune function and stress reduction; citrus fruit, tomatoes
	Vitamin D (ug/day)	5	10	15	5	10	15	Bone health; dairy, salmon, sunshine
	Vitamin E (mg/day)	15	15	15	15	15	15	Antioxidant; green leafy veggies
	Vitamin K (ug/day)	90	90	90	120	120	120	Soft tissue healing and liver function; green leafy veggies
	B1/Thiamin (mg/day)	1.1	1.1	1.1	1.2	1.2	1.2	Neurologic function; beef, pork
	B2/Riboflavin (mg/day)	1.1	1.1	1.1	1.3	1.3	1.3	Blood cell production; dairy products
	B3/Niacin (mg/day)	14	14	14	16	16	16	Lowers LDL and triglycerides, raises HDL; birds, fish, grain
	B5/Pantothenic A (mg/day)	5	5	5	5	5	5	Stress reduction; beans, meat, eggs, broccoli

SECTION 3: THRIVE MONTHS 3 AND 4

170

Sex		Women			Men			
Age		30-50	50-70	>70	30-50	50-70	>70	Function and Source
	Vitamin B6 (mg/day)	1.3	1.5	1.5	1.3	1.7	1.7	Protein metabolism and RBC function; potatoes, chicken, bananas
	B9/Folate (ug/day)	400	400	400	400	400	400	Blood flow, dissolves homocysteine; spinach, broccoli
	Vitamin B12 (ug/day)	2.4	2.4	2.4	2.4	2.4	2.4	Nerve function; seafood, fish
	Biotin (ug/day)	30	30	30	30	30	30	
	Cholin (mg/day)	425	425	425	550	550	550	
	Calcium (mg/day)	1000	1200	1200	1000	1200	1200	Bone health, increases HDL
	Iron (mg/day)	18	8	8	8	8	8	Oxygen transport in RBC; meat
	Phosphorus (mg/day)	700	700	700	700	700	700	Kidney and heart function, bone health; meat and dairy
	Iodine (ug/day)	150	150	150	150	150	150	
	Magnesium (mg/day)	320	320	320	420	420	420	Blood vessel health; green leafy vegetables
	Zinc (mg/day)	8	8	8	11	11	11	Antioxidant; meat, bird, seafood
	Selenium (ug/day)	55	55	55	55	55	55	Cancer protection; meat
	Copper (ug/day)	900	900	900	900	900	900	Antioxidant; nuts, beans
	Magnanese (mg/day)	1.8	1.8	1.8	2.3	2.3	2.3	Digestion and antioxidant; green leafy vegetables, coffee
	Chromium (ug/day)	25	20	20	35	30	30	

* Dietary reference intakes: Food and Nutrition Board, Institute of Medicine, National Academies.

HOW F.A.R. CAN YOU GO?

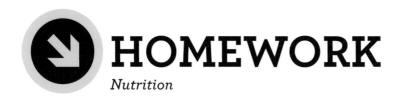

HOMEWORK
Nutrition

1. Continue using your food diaries. We will use them in the next section to calculate how many nutrients you consume.

2. List 10 most common carbs, proteins, and fats you eat.

3. List the grams in each food listed above. Compare what you are consuming to the daily recommendations.

4. What do you still need?

SECTION 3: THRIVE MONTHS 3 AND 4

NOTES

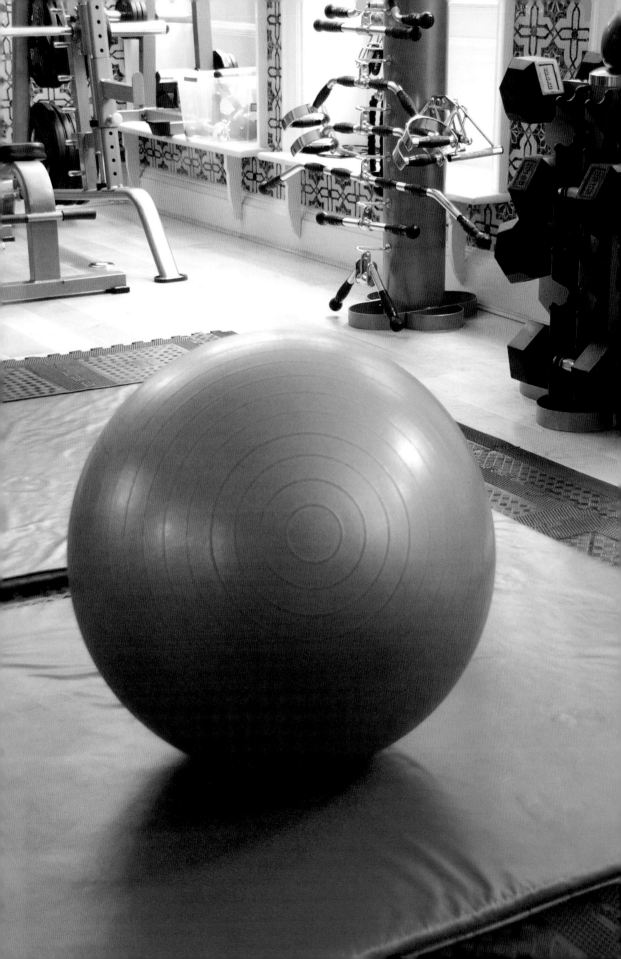

CHAPTER 11

Life, Liberty, and the Pursuit of Happiness

"Each morning when I open my eyes I say to myself, 'I, not events, have the power to make me happy or unhappy today. I can choose which it shall be. Yesterday is dead, tomorrow hasn't arrived yet. I have just one day, today, and I'm going to be happy in it.'"

—**Groucho Marx**

Well-being, contentment, life satisfaction, positive psychology, happiness, Bliss! No matter what we call it, pursuing Bliss is one of life's major preoccupations. Last year alone, more than 650 books about happiness were published. It's the subject of multiple magazine articles each month, and our very country was founded on the idea of pursuing life, liberty, and happiness.

Exactly what "happiness" is may be different for each of us, but researchers have identified what it is not. Happiness is not money. Researchers found people living near the poverty rate have happiness levels near those of people with means. This is because once your basic needs are met, more money does not buy you happiness.

Happiness does not belong to the young. As we age we accumulate a bank of happy memories that leads to contentment. A recent study by the Centers for Disease Control found that people in their twenties spend an average of 3.4 days per month feeling sad, while people in their seventies were sad only 2.3 days. Happiness apparently does not come from being smart, nor does it come from education.

What does make us happy includes things like a religious faith and friends. Researchers at the University of Illinois found the happiest people were the ones who spent the most time with friends and family. *Time* magazine surveyed Americans and found that 50 percent of us feel like we are living a very good or the best possible life most or all of the time; 80 percent of us generally wake up happy; and 79 percent of us consider ourselves optimistic. The top four things that make Americans happy are kids, family, faith, and spouse. Other mood elevators included listening to music, prayer, helping others, taking a bath, exercising, eating, taking a drive, and having sex.

However, happiness is not a constant high, according to Harvard professor Tal Ben-Shahar. In his popular Harvard class—more than 850 students take his class each semester—Dr. Ben-Shahar teaches, "Happiness is more than just a constant flow of positive emotions.... Happiness is a combination of meaning and pleasure."

Psychologists who study happiness describe it as a position, an overall characteristic or disposition. They believe it is possible to change our state of happiness by working at it, just like we change our bodies.

They also agree, however, that becoming happier is an active process. From finding that euphoric state we talked about after exercise to just acting happy when you do not necessarily feel that way, we tend to get happier. When I've gone through hard times, I've repeatedly told my friends that I choose to be happy, saying, "Our minds are stupid. If you just tell yourself you are happy, you will become a little more happy." The funny thing is that research bears this out. In the end, happiness begets happiness.

Scientists go a step further and encourage us to do the things we think will make us happy even if we don't feel like it. In other words, doing happy activities will make you happy. Dr. Sonja Lyubomirsky, author of *The How of Happiness*, contends that the pursuit of happiness is never done. "You can become happier just like you can become more fit. But you have to work at it every day of your life…. It's work, but the efforts work. It's not [always] fun trying to be grateful, optimistic, to invest in relationships, but at some point it will turn into a habit, a life-enhancing one."

▶ WANT TO KNOW HOW HAPPY YOU ARE?

While researching this book, I came across the University of Pennsylvannia's Authentic Happiness website (www.authentichappiness.sas.upenn.edu). The brainchild of Dr. Martin Seligman, the director of the University of Pennsylvania Positive Psychology Center, this site gives you free access to 19 questionnaires that gauge everything from your overall happiness, your current happiness, enduring happiness, character strength, and perseverance…you get the picture. Not only does it tell you how happy you are, it also tells you how happy you are compared to other people.

Go take a look, and take a test. It is fun, and you may learn something more about yourself.

What these psychologists are saying about working at happiness sounds a lot like what I have been saying about working on your bodies and brains. The remainder of this chapter continues with fun ways to work on your happiness, create your own space to de-stress your brain, and keep you brain sharp as you age.

▶ GET OFF THE COUCH

Somehow you knew I was going to say this. I will not be hurt if you go get a brain boost by putting down this book and going for an intense workout. Use one of the mini-circuits you learned in chapter 6 or 10, and fertilize your brain with a little sweat. On the other hand, why not maximize your benefit by putting this book on the book holder of a treadmill or elliptical and feed your brain while you give it something new to think about?

▶ GOOGLE YOUR BRAIN SMARTER

Studies have shown that when we Google, our brains make different neural connections than when we are reading a book. At least once per week, take a few minutes to learn about a subject you know nothing about on the Internet. Read for a few minutes, make the links, and learn a little. This is an excellent use for a couple minutes of "found time."

▶ COUNT YOUR BLESSINGS

University of California–Riverside psychologist Sonja Lyubomirsky found that keeping a gratitude journal and taking the time to count your blessings once per week significantly increased overall satisfaction with life. These kinds of exercises also raise energy levels, reduce pain, and decrease fatigue, especially if you elaborate more and have a wide span of things you are thankful for. Dr. Seligman also found that taking time to write down a trio of three blessings a day keeps us happy for more than six months.

So stop right now and count 10 of your blessings. Repeat this in detail each week for the next eight weeks.

1.

2.

3.

4.

5.

6.

7.

8.

9.

10.

Also, come up with a blessing trio each day.

1.

2.

3.

▶ DO A LITTLE SOMETHING NICE

Random acts of kindness refocus your energy outside yourself and provide a sense of satisfaction. The best "nice" thing to do for someone else is to simply thank them for doing something nice for you. Dr. Seligman found that paying a gratitude visit resulted in measurable increases in happiness for up to three months. Going further and doing for others, as in volunteering, adds to your sense of purpose.

▶ STOP TO NOTICE THE JOYS OF LIFE

I often tell my friends who are about to marry to take some time during the busy days surrounding the ceremony, and especially on their wedding day, to stand still and quietly observe all the joy swirling around them. I want them to lock in the memories and feelings and smells and excitements of the day instead of getting so caught up in the chaos that they can't remember the details of the moment.

In the same way, pay close attention to the moments of wonder and pleasure in your everyday life. Breathe deeply as you walk through the park in spring; stop and look at someone you love; pull your soft covers up and snuggle deep; sit back in your office and enjoy what you have accomplished; play your favorite music in the car on the way home, put your phone on vibrate, and sing loudly. There are plenty of joys in life if we take the time to stop and notice.

▶ LET GO

I have learned in life that holding on to anger only hurts me and not the person who hurt me in the first place. While I am ruminating on the wrong done to me and keeping my angst and blood pressure high, the other person often doesn't even know it. I'm the one who stays upset. I suggest you increase your well-being by letting go. It is a freeing choice. By doing so, the person who hurt you no longer has control over your emotions. Let go and forgive the person who hurt you. I'm not telling you to put yourself in a position to be hurt again. I'm suggesting you do yourself a mental and physical favor.

I feel the same way about the emotion of guilt. I believe the emotion of guilt is only productive if it spurs you, or the person who hurt you, into doing something about it. Simply feeling guilty without action allows us only to wallow in our wrongdoing, which doesn't help anyone. Take action to make it right, or stop luxuriating in a selfish emotion that doesn't help the person you hurt. Let go.

▶ DEEPEN RELATIONSHIPS

I suggested this in the first two months of your journey. How did deepening your personal relationships affect your happiness? Circle the wagons and keep a set of people close and connected to you. Reserve your tweets and texts for your fans.

▶ HAVE SEX

Nobel Prize-winning psychologist Daniel Kahneman of Princeton University studied more than 900 women, surveying them about the enjoyment of day-to-day activities and found that the five most positive activities for them were sex, socializing, relaxing, praying, and eating. Exercising was not far behind.

▶ CREATE WEEKLY "MY TIME"

This may seem like a stretch in our time-challenged world, but taking 30 minutes that are just your own can boost your energy for every other part of your life. This is not the time you invest in your workout—this is a few minutes where the phone is off, your mind is quiet, and you get to do something for yourself. Perhaps it is slow walk, a quick pedicure at the corner shop, tea at your favorite place, or a rendezvous with an old friend—anything that lets you disengage from the planning and delivery of life. I sometimes grab some of this when I'm on a plane. Instead of pulling out my computer for the hour flight to New York, I will buy a magazine full of pictures of beautiful things, people, and homes, then I grab a low-fat frozen yogurt and just spend the time quietly flipping pages and feeding my sweet tooth.

▶ DANCE AND SING

When was the last time you were silly? With my three-year-old, I am continuously silly, and I can tell you from recent experience that putting on loud music and dancing like crazy in the living room will leave you breathless, exhilarated, and laughing. It is an instant boost—try it!

CREATE A HOME SANCTUARY

While we can't always get away to the white sand beaches and relax—actually, I can't remember the last time I got away to a white-sand beach—we can create a bit of sanctuary right in our own homes to soothe our senses and melt away stress. Environmental psychologists studying sensory science believe that the environment you create can have a profound impact on your mood and attitude. Editors at *Prevention* suggest these ways for turning your home into your sanctuary:

1. Make your space touchable with corduroy and fleece. In studies, these fabrics made subjects feel content.

2. De-clutter your open spaces. Chaos makes you anxious, so the more you organize your space, the calmer you will feel. Literally, out of sight is out of mind.

3. Green up with plants and views outside to lower your blood pressure.

4. Use jasmine, hyacinth, cinnamon, and peppermint scents to lower stress and boost your mood.

5. Fill the room with music. Your ears know the difference between noise and sound.

6. Make your room roomy. Use mirrors, minimize furniture, and light the ceiling to expand the feel of your room.

▶ BRAIN SHARPENERS

Sometimes you may feel like you are losing your mind, but with age we are actually losing our brain. We can fight this loss of vital real estate with brain exercise. Look on the Internet and you will find an entire industry built around brain exercises. They focus on the five main areas of cognitive function—memory, attention, language, visual-spatial skills, and executive function. I suggest checking them out, downloading a few, and using a few minutes of your "found time" each day to sharpen your most vital organ.

Here are other simple ways to build your brain every day:

1. **Memorize the lyrics to new music.** Pop in a new tune every couple of days, and keep your brain hopping.

2. **Use your left hand.** I was born right-handed and started using my left hand to train my neuromuscular connections for surgery about 10 years ago. Now I'm nearly completely ambidextrous. Learning a new skill forces new neural connections. Yes, you really can teach an old dog new tricks.

3. **Change your routine.** When we get into a rut or routine, we use the same neural pathways over and over again. Simply change your daily routine, take another route home, or put your make-up on in a different order. This forces you to think through the process and re-engages your brain.

4. **Multitask.** To further break up your brain's habits, do several different activities at once. Read on the treadmill, listen to an educational CD in the car on the way home, jog a new route, etc.

5. **Learn a new language.** I'm not just talking about learning French and Italian here. I mean pick up a magazine on a subject you know nothing about and read a few articles. You will learn new vocabulary, pick up new information, and can share interesting new facts at your next cocktail party. If you are not into science, I suggest *Discover* magazine. I commonly pick up *Money*, *Forbes*, and *Architectural Digest*. I used to love the magazine *Best Life* by Rodale Press. I learned so much about what men are thinking.

6. **Get in your mind's eye.** Next time you walk into a new room, quickly look around and try to memorize what you see. When you leave, try to recall everything you saw, where it was located, who was there. If it is an interesting place, describe the scene in detail to your dinner partner. If you are a visual learner like I am, this might be easy for you. Personally, I have to really concentrate to remember what I hear. If you do too, then pay attention and try to remember everything about the next conversation you have.

7. **Reach out and say hello.** Social interactions force our brains to strategize, solve problems, and anticipate and consider options. All these activities are called the brain's "executive function."

You are going to have so much fun these two months building your Body, your Brains, and your Bliss. I think you see by now that THRIVE-ing is an Active process, and your best life is not lived sitting down. Stay the course in these two months. It's worth it. You are worth it!

▶ HOW HAPPY ARE YOU?

The founding father of happiness research, Edward Diener of the University of Illinois, devised this little scale to measure your Satisfaction with Life. It has been used by happiness researchers all over the world.

For the following five statements, use a 1–7 scale to rate your level of agreement:

1	2	3	4	5	6	7

Not at all true			Moderately true			Absolutely true

1. In most ways, my life is close to my ideal.

2. The conditions of my life are excellent.

3. I am satisfied with my life.

4. So far I have gotten the important things I want in life.

5. If I could live my life over, I would change almost nothing.

Scoring: 31-35 = Extremely satisfied with your life
26-30 = Very satisfied
21-25 = Slightly satisfied
20 = Neutral point
15-19 = Slightly dissatisfied
10-14 = Dissatisfied
5-9 = Extremely dissatisfied

LIFE, LIBERTY, AND THE PURSUIT OF HAPPINESS

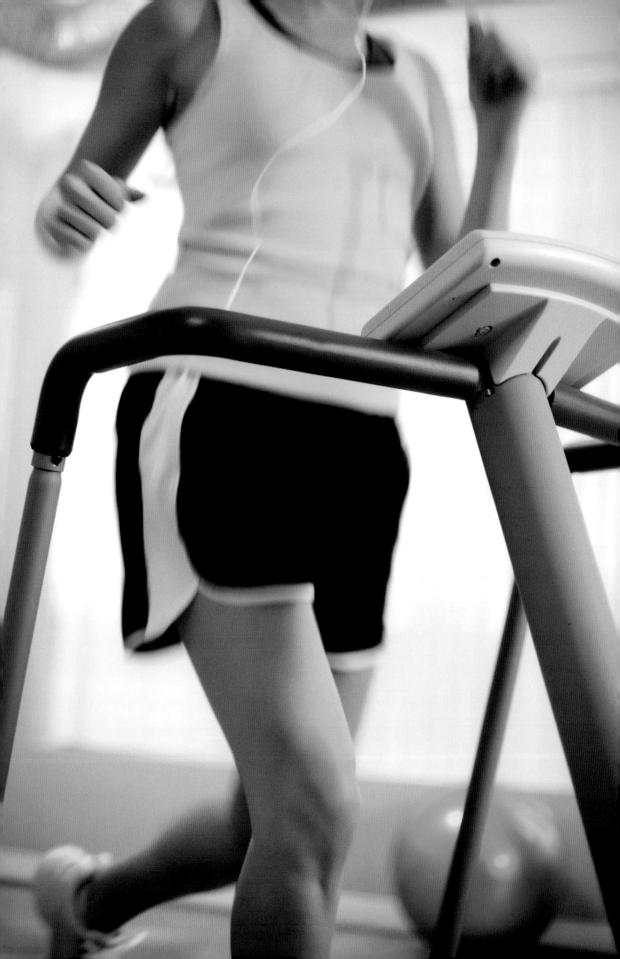

CHAPTER 12

Swagger!

*"Don't live down to expectations.
Go out there and do something remarkable."*
—Wendy Wasserstein

I hope that your four months of MOVE-ing, EAT-ing, THINK-ing, and FEEL-ing have given you an undeniable swagger. Walk tall, and be proud of what you have Achieved!

More good news is that your new muscle memory, brain power, and keys to happiness are not short-term gains. There is no finish line at the end of this book. You will always be different for having invested in yourself.

Before we continue this good life, pause here briefly and check your numbers. Ask your doctor to recheck any blood values that were abnormal when you started. Make a date with one of your accountability buddies, and talk about how you are doing. Shoot me a note at Vonda@vondawright.com. I want to hear about your experience!

Have you visited your THRIVE F.A.N. Club page lately? Go through your assessments again. Compare your health risk assessment data now with your original entries. Gathering real feedback about your progress is an important motivator for moving forward.

▶ **MOVE:** *Know Your Numbers*

	Two months	Four months	Comments
Weight			
Height			
Waist			Measure just below your naval. Ideally, women < 35 inches, men < 40 inches
Hip			Measure just above your hip bones
Waist/Hip Ratio (Divide your waist measurement by hip measurement)			Ideal is < 0.8, the closer to 1.0, the higher your health risks
Resting Heart Rate			Measure first thing in the morning or after sitting quietly for 15 minutes

	Two months	Four months	Comments
Obtain these values from a visit to your doctor's office			
Cholesterol			
Triglycerides			
LDL			
HDL			
Fasting Blood Glucose			
Blood Pressure			120/80 is normal
Percent Body Fat			

Take time to note how you are.

THRIV-ing:

1. How are you progressing toward the Vision of your future?

2. Have you taken Action by changing the way you Move and Eat? What is the best change you have made so far?

3. How is your Attitude after four months of THRIV-ing? Are you taking steps to build your Brian and increase your Bliss?

4. Because you are Achieving your goals…reward yourself today.

SECTION

④

THRIVE:
Months 5 and 6

"Go confidently in the direction of your dreams! Live the life you've imagined."

—Henry David Thoreau, *Walden*

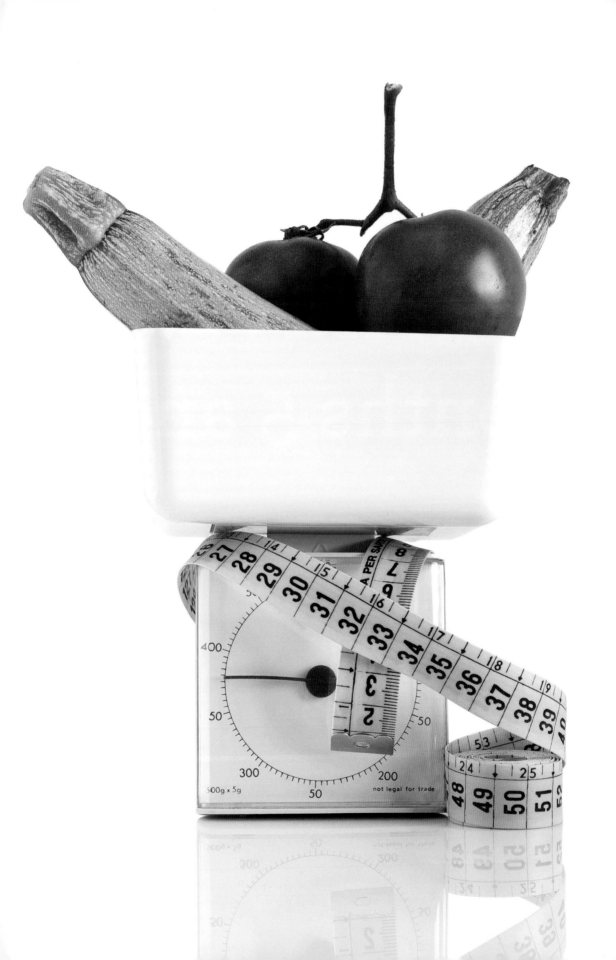

CHAPTER 13

This is the Year
I THRIVE

"You're off to Great Places!
Today is your day!
Your mountain is waiting,
So get on your way!"

— **Dr. Seuss,** *Oh, the Places You'll Go!*

What began as a Vision more than 16 weeks ago is snowballing into a THRIVE avalanche! Sometimes getting started is the hardest part. But once you are rolling, the momentum of your commitment to living a vital, active, joyful life takes over. You have lived a newer, richer experience, indeed.

The last section of this book is all about you taking over the THRIVE-ing process. Have you taken the Pizza Man's advice and figured out what is most important to you? What was your Vision when we started? Has it changed? What is your Vision going forward? What do you still have left to accomplish in order to THRIVE? What does it look like when you THRIVE?

▶ VISION-CAST FOR YOUR KIDS

A good friend of mine introduced me to the idea of Vision-casting for your children a few years before I had my daughter. He told me about a conversation he had with his high school junior about what she was really good at, what her interests were, what she wanted out of a college, and his hopes for her social development as she exited high school.

I was surprised that he would lay out his vision for her future in such great detail. But he reminded me that youth often have limited perspective and few experiences upon which to judge the outcomes of decision-making. He was not forcing her to follow his vision for her specifically; he was merely presenting all of the opportunities before her. I was fascinated with this idea, as I had often wished for specific guidance as I was growing up.

I have adopted the idea of Vision-casting even with my little one. I talk with her about all the possibilities—being an athlete, dancing on stage, singing opera, eating crème brulee in New York City, traveling on airplanes, running races, and so much more. I have taught her that the four steps to growing up big, strong, and happy are healthy food, exercise, sleep, and family. She has internalized these ideas. She wants to do them all, and she does. I'm vision-casting for her, showing her there is no limit.

▶ **ACTION:** *Show Me Your Own MOVE-s*

You have now reached a very exciting point in your MOVE toward THRIVE-ing—you are now ready to make your own MOVE-s! In the last four months, you have learned how to F.A.C.E. your future using total body circuits for F (flexibility), A (aerobic exercise), C (carrying a load), and E (equilibrium/balance). Your Body has gained strength and endurance, your Brain has learned more than 100 new exercises and made innumerable new neuromuscular connections, and the Bliss you feel from gaining confidence in your new skills and Body are undeniable. You have all the tools you need to create workouts just for you and THRIVE!

As you create your own workouts, here are some steps to guide you:

1. Look at the exercise summary table in chapter 10. Think about what worked for you, what you liked, and what you hated.

2. Identify your goal for the individual workout.

   a. Total Body THRIVE circuit?

   b. Focused THRIVE circuit for core, upper body/back, lower body?

   c. Aerobic workout?

   d. Aerobic + TBT stack?

3. Remember that your muscles and brain love intensity and variety. They will get stronger and more efficient if you mix up your workouts every week. Also remember that as long as you are covering the major muscle groups each week, your muscles will be happy.

4. You can plan your workout schedule a day, a week, or even a month in advance.

5. Don't forget to incorporate F (flexibility) and E (equilibrium/balance) into your everyday routine.

▶ SAMPLE WORKOUT STRUCTURE

TBT Circuit

This short but intense workout pattern gets your whole body MOVE-ing.

1. Choose 10 TBT exercises from your menu.

2. Include moves that focus on each body part, for instance:

   a. Two for your core.

   b. Two for your upper body.

   c. Two for your lower body.

   d. Two for your buttocks.

   e. Two aerobic/pliometrics.

3. After warming up with a five-exercise dynamic warm-up circuit of your choice, perform each TBT move for 45 seconds, alternating with 15 seconds of rest.

4. Each circuit repetition will take approximately 10 minutes.

5. Your goal is three complete circuits, or 30 minutes of work.

Focused Pairs Workout

Pairing opposing body parts in a workout pattern is an amazing way to jack up the intensity and be efficient with your time.

1. Plan these workouts a week at a time to ensure you pay attention to each region at least twice a week.

2. Decide which areas you will pair.

   a. Core/upper body

   b. Core/lower body

   c. Upper body/lower body

3. Select five TBT exercises for each body part to create the circuit.

4. After warming up with a five-exercise dynamic warm-up circuit of your choice, perform each TBT move for 45 seconds, alternating with 15 seconds of rest.

5. Each circuit repetition will take approximately 10 minutes.

6. Your goal is three complete circuits, or 30 minutes of work.

Aerobic Circuits

I don't have to tell you that doing the same aerobic workout every day can get really boring, whether you are on the road, the treadmill, or on a bike. Why not throw in an aerobic circuit once in a while? This takes a little logistical planning, but it is fun and intense. This is Powerplay.

1. In your health club or home gym, identify the various pieces of aerobic equipment you want to use. Each is a station.

2. Plan your route.

3. After warming up with a five-exercise dynamic warm-up circuit of your choice, spend three to four minutes on each apparatus alternating with a one-minute recovery, then move to the next station.

    a. Four minutes on treadmill at 70–80 percent maximum intensity.

    b. One-minute recovery, then move to next station.

    c. Four minutes at 70–80 percent on spin bike.

    d. One-minute recovery, then move to next station.

    e. Four minutes of jump rope.

    f. One-minute recovery, then move to the next station.

    g. Four minutes on the rowing machine.

    h. One-minute recovery, then move to the next station.

4. Perform one to two circuits through the stations depending on how long your target time is.

5. This circuit can also be performed outside on a track if you place your street bike at your starting point and substitute four minutes of pliometrics for the rowing machine.

Aerobic Stacks

As you have learned, these aerobic stacks pair an A (aerobic) workout with a C (carrying a load) workout. You can stack them any way you want:

1. Five TBT exercises (2–3 complete circuits) followed by 30 minutes of AE.

2. Aerobic/TBT intervals:

    a. Two-minute AE (any method you choose).

    b. One-minute TBT exercise.

      c. Two-minute AE.

      d. One-minute TBT.

      e. Continue to alternate two-minute AE with one-minute TBT for 30–45 minutes.

    4. As always, to avoid injury, warm up with a five-move dynamic warm-up circuit.

▶ MOVE WITH FRIENDS AND FAMILY

Throughout this book, I keep talking about how MOVE-ing your Body is not only work but also a lot of fun. In fact, I believe you have to enjoy it in order to stick with it. Did you know, however, that exercising in groups of friends or family is actually better for your Brain? Your neurons really get fired up when you add social contact to exercise. Research out of Princeton University found that when animals getting off the couch for the first time (figuratively, of course) are exercised in groups, they made more neurons than if they exercised in isolation. This is because beginning an exercise program is stressful and can induce stress hormones. The social support of a group you are comfortable in seems to minimize the stress and maximize the benefit of exercise on your brain.

Another reason for activating your family and friends is that by saving their mobility, you are actually saving their lives. I am passionate about this. As household leaders and health-care decision-makers, you are in a powerful position to change the lives of those you care most about. By now, your friends and family have noticed you are THRIVE-ing. They are probably commenting to you about the changes in your Body and Attitude. Now that you have their attention, invite them to join you. Believe me, they are inspired by and proud of your progress.

If your friends and family are already MOVE-ing regularly, challenge them to join you for a TBT circuit or Aerobic Stack. Make it a game. Make if fun. You will strengthen your body and your relationship.

If your friends and family are stepping away from the couch for the first time in years, invite them to join you for a mini-TBT circuit from chapter 6 and a walk. Remember how it was to start out four months ago, and teach them a little at a time to THRIVE. Make it a game. Make it fun. You may save their lives.

▶ TEACH YOUR CHILDREN TO THRIVE

I encourage you to teach the children in your life how to MOVE. Whether they are your own children, your nieces and nephews, or the neighbors' kids, they are watching you and learning from every move you make.

The sad truth is that in this country we have an epidemic of overweight and sedentary children. Their bodies are old before their time, and they are living with chronic metabolic diseases previously seen in old age. Our children are overweight and immobile largely because we teach them to be that way. Research shows that the children of overweight and sedentary parents have an 80 percent higher likelihood of being overweight and sedentary themselves. They are watching and learning from us. If they are not moving, it is because we have taught them not to.

The good news is that they will watch and learn from us while we're moving, too. It's easy. Their little bodies are designed to MOVE, and they want to be like us. Think of toddlers with boundless energy running all over the place. By teaching them to do what you are doing, you are strengthening their bodies, enlarging their brains, and paving the way for their futures.

I have an amazing three-year-old running around my house right now. I'm in awe that when I get down on the floor with a foam roller she grabs her little yellow foam roller and rolls away with me. She has raced with me since her first birthday when I carried her through a 5k race in her little Baby Bjorn. Now she regularly helps me "teach" my marathon cross-training classes. It is so much fun. We are spending time together, and she is learning that to grow up strong and healthy takes exercise and good food. Just ask her—she'll tell you.

▶ PLANNING AHEAD TO EAT WELL

In your first two months of THRIVE-ing, you learned to gain control over food by learning about your EAT-ing habits, how to make simple substitutions, and the 500 Rule. In the last two months, you learned about food—Nutrition 101, if you will. Nutrition is complex and sometimes frustrating, but the more you know, the better choices you can make. We are all capable of eating well; it is not magic, but I understand that sometimes it is hard.

If you read my first book, *Fitness After 40*, you may remember the story I told about eating as a surgical resident. Those bad habits resulted in a slow accumulation of 20 pounds. In general, residents eat whatever and whenever they can (including that hours-old pizza left in the surgical lounge) because they are never sure when they will have time to eat again. Sometimes residents eat out of a need to pamper the feeling of self-pity that comes when you are working at 3:00 AM when everyone else you know is asleep in their beds. This pattern of eating was a hard habit to break even when my schedule became more tolerable. I broke this bad EAT-ing cycle by knowing myself, knowing my food, and planning ahead.

You may feel like a surgical resident in your busy life, grabbing a quick bite whenever it fits into your day, and you may feel too tired to make a healthy meal after you get home. Here are tips for planning ahead to EAT well.

1. **Keep it simple.** We all love the 20-ingredient, multi-flavor, succulent dishes. Unfortunately these usually require immense prep time. Reserve these luxuries for the weekends, and keep your mid-week food simple and stress free.

2. **Avoid any food that is not a primary color.** Plants and animals grow in primary colors, while processed foods can come in any color imaginable.

3. **Eat stand-alone foods.** To know exactly what you are eating, eat foods that stand alone. It is hard to know exactly what is in a casserole or cream soup, etc. On the other hand, if you are eating a pile of green beans, you know you are eating a pile of green beans.

4. **Keep healthy snacks in your desk or purse.** You are more likely to avoid running to the vending machine if you have a little something near at hand to kill those afternoon cravings.

To give you an idea of how to keep your mid-week dinners simple, I wrote down what I fed my family last week. Although I love to cook, I am tired and hungry when I get home and I don't want to spend all night in the kitchen.

Here is what I do to plan ahead to EAT well:

1. Limit mid-week meal menus to three to four stand-alone foods that cover all of the Macro-nutrients:
   a. Protein/fat from meat
   b. Carbs in the form of pasta, grain, potatos, etc.
   c. Primary-colored fruits and vegetables
2. Limit preparation time to 30 minutes.
3. When roasting or broiling, line all pans in the oven with foil to minimize clean-up.
4. Keep your kitchen stocked with stand-alone foods so you can mix and match without a recipe.

Dinner last week in the Wright house, which was on the table in 30 min or less:

Monday

Arctic char filet: Brush entire filet with a small amount of olive oil, salt, and pepper to taste, then broil for 5–10 minutes until desired consistency.

Peapods: Wash and eat raw or sautéed until just tender.

Bell peppers: Cut in half, brush with small amount of olive oil, and broil with char.

Couscous: Five-minute prep per box instructions.

Strawberries: Wash and go.

➜TIPS

Minimize calories by keeping total olive oil use to 1 Tablespoon.

Minimize prep time by putting on couscous water to boil, preparing the char and peppers and putting them in the broiler, then sautéing peapods and finishing couscous while char is broiling.

I always keep strawberries and pineapple on hand for my sweet tooth after dinner.

Tuesday

Chicken breast: Tenderized with mallet, added salt and pepper to taste, then sautéed in nonstick grill pan.

Broccoli crowns: Boiled with cube of chicken bullion for taste.

Brown rice

Vonda's Usual Salad

TIPS

Tenderizing chicken makes it tender and minimizes cooking time.

Broccoli is amazing plain—no cheese required!

Put the rice on to cook first, as it takes the longest to complete.

Prepare a big salad ahead of time and keep it in the refrigerator to eat at any time.

Vonda's Usual Salad
Mache
Cucumbers
Roasted beets
Grape tomatoes
Portabello mushrooms
Balsamic vinaigrette or olive oil and lemon juice

Wednesday

I teach a marathon cross-training program on Wednesdays, so we were in and out the door again.

Turkey and light Swiss cheese sandwiches on wheat bread with lettuce and tomatoes (No mayo!)

Vonda's Usual Salad

Carrot sticks

Whole fruit

Thursday

Alaskan salmon: Brush with a small amount of olive oil, salt and pepper to taste, then broil seven to 10 minutes

Spinach linguine: Tossed lightly in garlic-infused olive oil

Sautéed asparagus spears: No sauce!

Roasted tomato halves

TIPS

Put water on to boil for linguine first.

Prep salmon and tomato halves and put in oven.

Limit total olive oil use to minimize calories.

Friday

Flank steak: Salt and pepper to taste, cook to medium rare.

Roasted sweet or yellow potatoes sliced to 1/8 inch and roasted in oven

Roasted cauliflower: Cut into florets, toss in baggie with olive oil, salt, and pepper, then roast/broil in oven. This prep condenses the flavor.

Sautéed spinach

Glass of pinot noir

Nutrition Facts for a Week in the Wright House

	Portion	Protein (g)	Carbs (g)	Fat (g)	Calories	Extras
Monday						
Char	4 oz.	24	0	8	204	
Coucous	2 oz.	8	43	1	221	Fiber
Pea pods	1 cup	8	21	1	117	Vitamins C, K
Bell peppers	1 cup	1	9	0	46	Fiber, Vitamins C, A
Olive oil	1 Tbs.				100	Omega 3, Omega 6
Strawberries	1 cup	1	12	0	49	Fiber, Vitamin C
Tuesday						
Chicken breasts	4 oz.	24	0	1	124	Niacin, B6
Broccoli	1 cup	3	6	0	31	Vitamins C, K, A
Brown rice	1 cup	5	46	2	218	Fiber, manganese
Wednesday						
Turkey	2 oz.	8	4	0	62	
Wheat bread	2 slices	8	24	4	138	fiber
Romaine Lettuce	½ cup	½	1	0	4	Vitamins A, K, C
Tomato	1 large	2	7	0	33	Lycopene, Vitamins C, K, A
Carrot sticks	1 cup	1	12	0	52	Vitamin A
Apple	1	0	25	0	95	Fiber
Thursday						
Alaskan salmon	4 oz.	24	0	8	172	B12, Omega 3
Spinach linguini	1 cup	8	43	1	221	Fiber
Asparagus	1 cup	3	5	0	27	Vitamin K, Folate
Roasted tomatoes	1 large	2	7	0	33	
Friday						
Flank steak	4 oz.	24	0	9	186	Niacin, B6
Roasted potatoes	1 cup	2	26	0	104	Fiber, Vitamin C
Cauliflower	1 cup	2	5	0	25	Fiber, Vitamin C
Sautéed spinach	1 cup raw	1	1	0	7	Vitamins K, A
Pinot noir					124	Reseritrol

▶ BONE HEALTH NUTRITION

As an orthopedic surgeon, I spend my life thinking about bone health and making these architectural wonders as strong as they can be. For the strongest bones, you need to "bash" them. By this I mean stress them with impact exercise, such as walking, running, jumping, etc. In addition, bones also stay stronger when they are surrounded by powerful muscles to dampen the load and move them through a range of motions.

Bones are dynamic and growing I-beams that not only keep us upright but serve as the major metabolic storehouse of our bodies. Therefore we must feed them. By now you know your bones need calcium to maintain strength and Vitamin D to absorb the calcium from your gut, but your bones need more than that.

Calcium

Whole foods outperform supplements as a source of most bone-healthy nutrients. Make selections that contain more than 10 percent of the daily value. Many foods are now fortified with calcium, making it easier to accumulate what we need. Look for these items:
- ✓ **Milk, yogurt, cheese**
- ✓ **Orange juice fortified with Vitamin C**
- ✓ **Cereals fortified with Vitamin C**
- ✓ **Dark green leafy veggies, such as kale, broccoli, spinach**
- ✓ **Seafood, such as oysters, perch, clams, blue crab, shrimp.**

When you can't get enough, and most of us can't, calcium supplements are mandatory for bone health. Calcium supplements come in two varieties—calcium carbonate, and calcium citrate. Bones don't care which kind you take, just as long as you do. They must be taken differently, however. Calcium carbonate should be taken with meals because they need stomach acid to absorb. Calcium citrate doesn't need to be taken with food. In general, you absorb more calcium when these supplements are taken with food and when no more than 500 mg are taken at one time. Most of these supplements also come in formulas that include a dose of vitamin D. If you get the combination form, you'll get both nutrients in one pill.

Vitamin D

Calcium cannot do its job without Vitamin D opening the door to let it out of the gut and into the body. Vitamin D comes from the sun, but anyone living north of Atlanta doesn't get enough sunshine each day to make enough. So look for milk fortified with Vitamin D; fish, such as salmon, tuna, and sardines; and other fortified foods.

Other Important Nutrients for Bone Health

There are a few other nutrients needed for bones:
- ✓ **Phosphorus: dairy, yogurt**
- ✓ **Protein: meat, diary, yogurt**
- ✓ **Vitamin A: fish, dark green leafy vegetables, citrus fruit, cheese, eggs**
- ✓ **Vitamin B12: meat, fish, eggs, fortified cereal**
- ✓ **Vitamin C: essential for collagen formation. Collagen is the scaffold that bones are built on. Foods rich in Vitamin C include broccoli, bell peppers, cauliflower, kale, lemons, strawberries**
- ✓ **Vitamin K: broccoli, brussel sprouts, cabbage, olive oil, spinach**

▶ MUSCLE HEALTH NUTRITION

According to a survey developed by Abbott Labs and the AGS Foundation for Health in Aging, nine out of 10 people think that feeling weaker is the worst part of aging. Despite this, many people are not taking the critical steps to ensure their more than 650 muscles remain strong and healthy. Clinical research shows that starting at age 40, we begin to lose 8 percent of our muscle mass per decade. This loss rises to 15 percent by our seventh decade, which can lead to weakness, falls, low energy, and fat accumulation.

In addition to C (carrying a load) with the TBT exercises in your arsenal, you must focus on nutrition for strong muscles.

Protein

Muscles are made of protein, and their building blocks are the amino acids. When you use your muscles in daily activity or exercise, they are broken down. But protein repairs this damage and rebuilds muscle. Eat protein at every meal beginning with breakfast. Good sources include meat, chicken, fish, eggs, beans, and dairy products.

Vitamins and Minerals

Calcium, magnesium, potassium, and phosphorous are important nutrients that ensure muscles contract as they should. This is especially true for the heart.

Vitamin C aids in the formation of collagen and elastin, which are important for the elasticity and flexibility of muscles. In addition, Vitamin C is a powerful antioxidant that repairs the micro-tears our muscles sustain during hard exercise sessions.

Vitamin E is another proven muscle-rebuilding antioxidant and can diminish delayed onset muscle soreness.

▶ BRAIN HEALTH NUTRITION

Socked away from the rest of the body in its high and mighty position, the brain is in charge of everything we do. It deserves all the special attention we can give it. Just as exercise can improve brain function and growth, nutrition is key for both Brains and Bliss!

Water

The brain is about 80 percent water, so keep it tanked up with water. Dehydration increases the brain's stress levels and affects thinking.

Fish Oil

Our brains are also made of fat—fatty acids, that is. DHA, one form of Omega 3 fatty acids, makes up much of the brains' gray manner and neurons. Dietary Omega 3 from fish or plants is vital for optimal thinking.

Antioxidants

Dietary antioxidants—such as green tea, dark chocolate, resveratrol, fruits, and dark green leafy vegetables—counter the development of toxic ions in the brain called free-radicals, which contribute to cognitive deterioration with age. The best antioxidant fruits and veggies include blueberries, blackberries, cranberries, strawberries, spinach, raspberries, brussels sprouts, plums, broccoli, beets, avocados, oranges, red grapes, red bell peppers, cherries, and kiwis. Vitamins A and C are also powerful antioxidants.

Vitamin B

Many B vitamins are vital to normal brain and nerve function. Most of the B vitamins, as well as folic acid, have specific advantages for your brain and nervous system:

✓ **Vitamin B1 (Thiamine):** Essential for healthy brain and nerve cells.

✓ **Vitamin B5 (Pantothenic acid):** Forms a coenzyme that helps in transmission of nerve impulses.

✓ **Vitamin B6 (Pyridoxine):** Helps convert tryptophan into serotonin, a brain chemical.

✓ **Vitamin B12 (Cyanocobalamin):** Helps maintain healthy nervous tissue. It is found in eggs, meat, fish, and poultry, as well as milk and dairy products.

✓ **Folic acid:** Essential for metabolism of long-chain fatty acids in the brain. It is found in bananas, orange juice, fortified cereals, lemons, strawberries, cantaloupe, leafy vegetables, dried beans, and peas. It is especially important for pregnant women because low levels increase the risk of neural tube defects in newborns.

My job as a teacher and doctor is to equip you to THRIVE on your own. Are you ready to MOVE and EAT on your own? Definitely. Continue to use the THRIVE F.A.N. Club every month as a tool to track your individual fitness and nutrition data, stay updated on my website, www.vondawright.com, and live the life you envisioned.

▶ ATTITUDE

I hope you have experienced the profound connection between your Body, Brains, and Bliss during the last 16 weeks. As your Body grew strong, so did your Brain, and you have gained a new perspective for future Bliss.

What follows are some of my favorite ways of challenging my Brains and pursuing Bliss.

1. **Meet inspirational people.** I like to talk to people at the top of their fields about their paths, how they did it, why they became interested in what they do, what their vision was, and more. I want to know what it was like along the way, what it felt like. It is not only fascinating, but it also gives me a lot to think about.

2. **Learn from your patients.** Okay, I know not all of you have patients, but the point is learn from people you come in contact with. Whenever I see patients for the first time, I note what they do for a living. Often at the end of a visit I will ask them about their profession. I'm curious, I learn a lot, and it gives me a deeper understanding of who the person I'm caring for is. By doing this, I have learned about high-performance tires, mining the Marcella Shale for natural gas in Pennsylvania, landscaping, finance and investing, amazing travel destinations, and the best places in Pittsburgh to get kids' stuff. You can learn from anybody. Take advantage of it.

3. **Make a THRIVE bucket list.** The first person I knew who actually had a bucket list was an unfortunate friend of mine who broke his back when he was 18 and had to spend several months immobile waiting for it to heal. He used that time to Vision-cast about his future, although I'm not sure he knew that's what he was doing. He made a bucket list for his life, filling it with all kinds of lofty and practical goals, such as own my own business, create a million bucks before I'm 30, write a book, marry, and travel the world with my wife.

   I wrote a THRIVE bucket list filled with mostly right-brain, out-of-the-box life experiences. They are meant to inspire my mostly left-brained rational life. On my list, I included hike Macchu Picchu (I did), be in an opera (I was in two), write books (I have), create deep and abiding friendships (I work on it daily), go to the Moto GP superbike races (I did, and there is something sexy about 170 mph!), attend Mercedes Fashion Week (I did as a guest of Mercedes), and cultivate a national platform on sports medicine and active aging (in progress). Plus I have so many more dreams still left to fulfill, such as go to Millionaire's Row at the Kentucky Derby, watch a NASCAR race from pit row, be on the sideline at the Super Bowl, live in Tuscany with my family for a summer, take Italian cooking classes, set up my family financially, travel with my family to a new country every year, explore the West with my daughter…. The list goes on and on. These dreams add flavor and inspiration to my life.

4. **Enter a competition.** I'm not necessarily talking about a road race, but you can enter anything that challenges you—a

bake-off, a chess tournament, whatever. The physical challenge coupled with the problem-solving of navigating a big race and the adrenaline rush of hard work is a sure-fire way to THRIVE.

5. **Get more sleep.** We need a cycle of rest daily. Optimally that cycle should be 7½ hours. I can tell you as one of the last doctors to train without work-hour restrictions that you cannot underestimate the value of sleep for your health and sense of well-being.

▶ ACHIEVE

You have come so far, but this is no time to rest on your laurels. Actually, I view this as the beginning. You are strong, smart, happy, and in control.

Celebrate what you have Achieved by throwing yourself a THRIVE party. Choose a day near the end of this six months. Invite your circle of friends, the ones you talked through your Vision-planning with, the ones who hit the road with you and anyone who knew about this ride. Get a new outfit to show off what your MOVEs have done for you. Plan a great meal highlighting how you learned to EAT. Spend the evening telling stories, bragging, and celebrating your hard work.

Write and tell me about your THRIVE stories. Send me pictures of your THRIVE parties. I want to share in your joy, experience your Bliss, and celebrate the new swagger in your life. I'm proud of you. I'm honored and thankful that you invested time in yourself by investing time with me.

These are the best years.

This is the year you will THRIVE!

APPENDIX I

Guide to THRIVE at Your Fingertips

Use your smart phone to connect instantly with "Dr. Vonda Wright's Guide to THRIVE."

APPENDIX II

Some of Dr. Wright's Favorite Online Sites

The Internet is packed with an abundance of information for maximizing your Body, Brain, and Bliss connection. Here are a few sites that I keep track of regularly:

www.vondawright.com This is my own website where you can find my latest programs, blogs, products, and recommendations.

www.sharecare.com Dr. Oz's health information website where the answers to any medical question you have are expertly provided by some of this country's prominent physicians and fitness experts.

www.fitstudio.com A great resource for fitness and nutrition programs.

www.nsga.com This member of the Olympic committee governs the National Summer Senior Games, the Senior Olympics, for athletes ages 50 and above.

www.aaos.org American Academy of Orthopaedic Surgeons

www.sportsmed.org American Orthopaedic Society for Sports Medicine

www.icaa.cc International Council on Active Aging

www.whineat9.com MaryLou Quinlin and Dr. Nancy Berk's weekly podcast where you will laugh out loud about whatever is bugging you and turn problems into solutions.

www.marathonshow.com The Marathon Show with Joe Taricani is a radio show dedicated to marathon runners and marathons.

www.moremagazine.com

www.runnersworld.com A great resource for runners of all ages and skill levels.